This book should be returned to any branch of the
Lancashire County Library on or before the date

urself
URAL

Dedication

For Evie – my lotions and potions girl.

OVER 50 EASY-TO-MAKE HOMEMADE REMEDIES GATHERED FROM NATURE

treat yourself
NATURAL

Sof McVeigh
Foreword by
Kirstie Allsopp

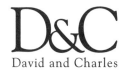

D&C
David and Charles

Contents

Foreword by Kirstie Allsopp   06

Introduction   08

Plants   10

Techniques   12

Basic Kit   16

Spring	18
Summer	46
Autumn	76
Winter	106
Glossary	136
Acknowledgements/About the Author	138
Useful Books	140
Directory	141
Index	142

Foreword by Kirstie Allsopp

This is not a coffee table book – I've never really understood that concept anyway – when I buy a book I want to learn something from it, within weeks I want it to be slightly grubby from use, and this is just such a book. It is practical, straightforward and easy to use. Sof is a great friend of mine and an inspiration; her understanding of a hedgerow and how its treasures can be husbanded is extraordinary.

I know that making things yourself has enormous benefits, but making things from the fields or your garden, which you can then use on your skin, feed to your friends and family or keep your blankets moth-free seems to be doubly beneficial.

This book is full of brilliant ideas for things to make for yourself, or as wonderful gifts. Year in year out this will be an invaluable resource for a rainy day or a country walk, written by someone who really knows what she is talking about as well as living the same busy life as you and I.

x x x

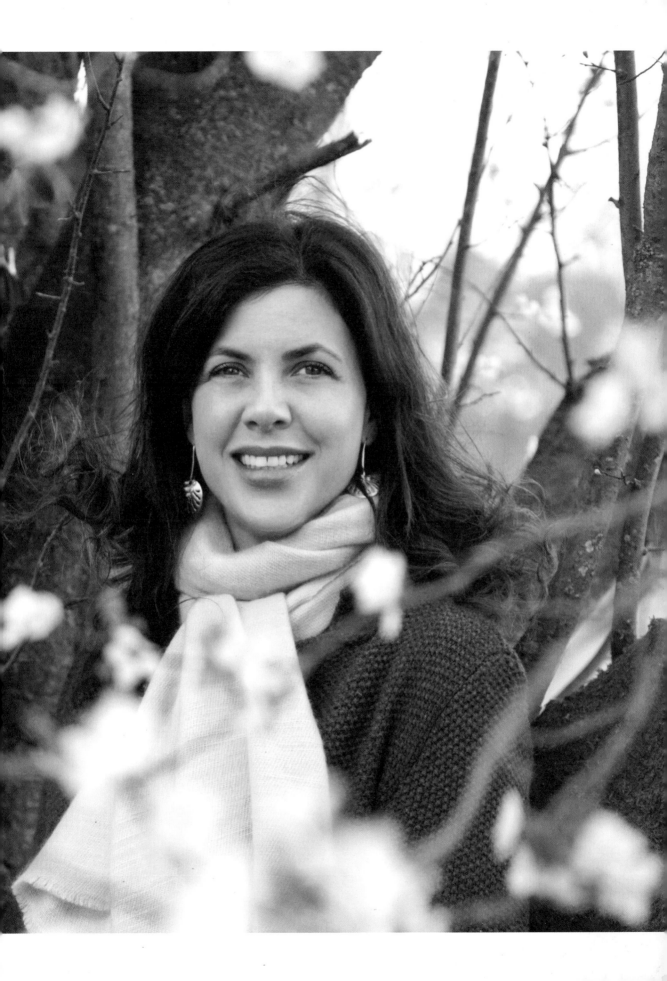

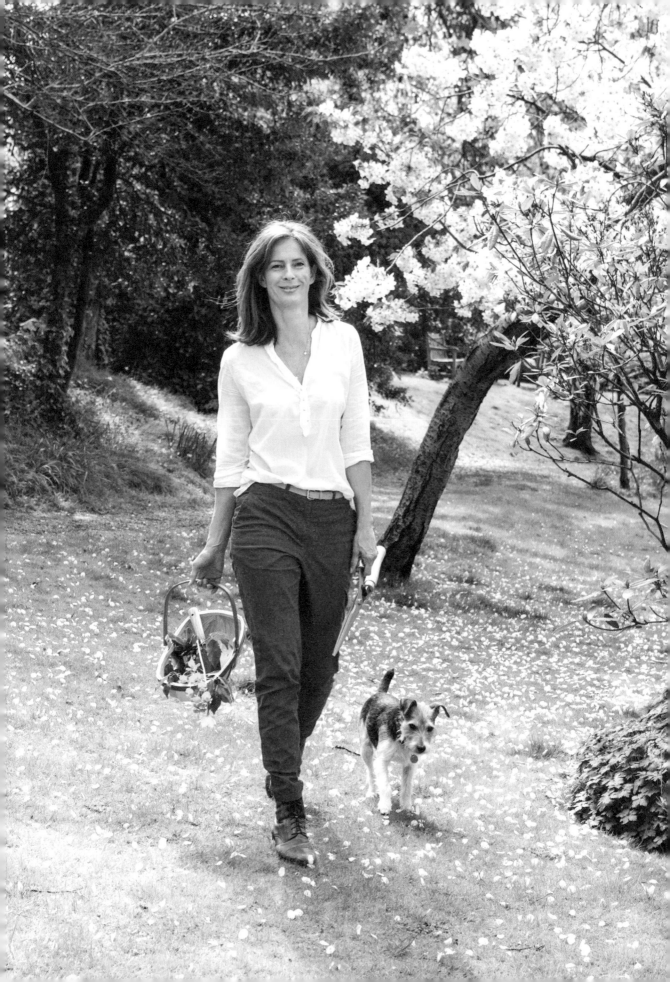

Introduction

Within this book I hope you will discover how easy it is to harness the natural goodness of plants that can help us feel better, look better and have a healthy year. Sprinkled throughout you'll find lashings of common sense and a splash of fun, seasoned with a healthy love of nature and all that it can offer us. Not to mention many wonderful and easy recipes, so you can see just what Mother Nature has in her store cupboard.

I think creating things is hard-wired into us, whether this may be making a delicious meal, writing a song or painting a beautiful picture; making something leaves us with a sense of contentment that is hard to beat. I love making things but I know how busy all our lives can be, so these recipes are simple and straightforward, enabling you to achieve maximum results with a great sense of satisfaction – yet you won't have to spend all day on them.

A large part of this book is about using plants that are readily available – or free, such as nettles, dandelions and hawthorn berries. I hope it will encourage you to get out there and to keep your eyes open, so you can discover the many widely available plants that you can use for your health – with the added bonus that they're not costing you anything.

With this in mind I have laid the book out 'Season by Season', so you will know at a glance what to gather and when to gather it. So in the bountiful spring months you can pick abundant fresh leaves, in the summer it's the pretty flowers, then in autumn comes lush berries and hips. Even in the cold, quiet winter months there are bulbs and evergreen herbs to use.

Within each season you'll find useful tips on using nature for your wellbeing relevant to that season. So in summer there are ideas about travelling, and in winter there are suggestions on what you can do to beat the common cold. In autumn I cover burns as it's the bonfire season, and in spring I touch on the benefits of bees and their produce as they sleepily re-emerge.

I hope you will feel empowered to explore the wonderful world of making remedies, either for yourself or as gifts for your friends and family; I think there is nothing nicer than a lovingly made homemade present. Some gift ideas you'll find in here include ginger chocolates, lavender bath salts and, for some lip-licking goodness, try making the chocolate lip balms.

Or just treat yourself to a soothing chamomile bath, followed by a rose oil body balm; what else could be more relaxing? Why don't you give it a go, and while soaking in the bath, see what other remedies you'd like to make. I think you'll be surprised at just how easy they are and how much fun you'll have.

Plants

In every culture across the world you will find a long history of using plants for health and wellbeing, and many of the common medicines we use today are derived from them. This is because plants contain many active compounds and chemicals known as phytochemicals: some of these are beneficial to our health, some are not, and others are poison. Moreover, different parts of a plant can contain different phytochemicals: so the root of a plant could be used for one thing, the berries of the same plant for another, while the leaves may have no use at all.

Most of the plants I have chosen for this book are common and plentiful, so it is easy to forage for them, like dandelions and nettles. Others are well known plants and easily available, like mint and lavender. I have also included a few berries that you can gather, such as the classic blackberry and the abundant elderberry. Finally, there are a few less recognizable plants, like lemon verbena or lady's mantle; these are easy to grow and make lovely additions to a garden or a windowsill.

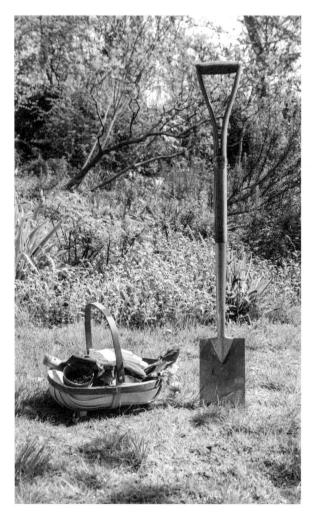

TO GARDEN OR NOT TO GARDEN

Over the past 10 years I have become an avid gardener in order to grow a ready supply of plants from which to create my natural remedies. I enjoy the cycle of nature, marvelling at its resilience and its ability to bounce back from whatever is thrown at it. Nature will tell you what will work in your garden, not the other way round, and I love this refusal on the part of nature to be controlled. I garden organically, so using weeds comes naturally to me – I actually have rather a lot of these in my garden!

If you like gardening, I recommend keeping a small patch of your garden for healing plants grown specifically for treatments. I've created my own area – grandly naming it my Medicinal Garden – in Devon in south-west England; this has been a great source of information on plants, along with a hefty dose of trial and error. Some plants have flourished, such as pot marigold and chamomile; some have taken over, such as wormwood; while some have not fared so well, like my rather sad-looking arnica.

If you are not a gardener don't worry, most of the plants in this book can be found on common ground where you can forage for them (see Foraging) or most of the herbs can be bought in pots in supermarkets. For the other plants, a trip to a local garden centre is a good idea, or you can buy dry herbs from most health stores.

FORAGING

Over the past few years, the pastime of foraging for plants has slowly been gaining momentum – a welcome return to the human hunter-gatherer instincts that must be deeply rooted somewhere within all of us; the process connects us with nature in an almost primeval way.

If you are not sure how to start foraging, try joining a foraging group in your local area – they are springing up all over the place. Or just go for a walk, with a good guidebook and a knowledgeable friend to provide advice. Once you start looking around, you'll be amazed at just how much you do recognize; try foraging first for blackberries then build your confidence from there. With a good lashing of common sense, nature's bounty can be yours for the taking.

When I say 'for the taking', I do mean within reason: all good foragers respect nature. They know not to over-pick or over-gather, always leaving some for the bees and birds, as well as enough to regenerate the plant again for another year. At the same time, with certain plants such as the rose and elderflower, you will not want to pick too many flowers in the Spring or you will not be able to harvest the hips and berries in the Autumn.

In our far more urbanized and intensively farmed landscape there are undoubtedly fewer wild areas, so share what you find and leave more for another year. If you are gathering plants or berries to use in the recipes in this book, please be absolutely certain you know what you are picking; there is no room for trial and error, and alongside nature's goodies, there are also many poisonous plants and berries. The golden rule of foraging applies at all times:

'IF IN DOUBT, THEN LEAVE IT OUT'

HOMEOPATHY

Homeopathy has been in use since the eighteenth century, and is based on the principle of treating 'like with like'. This means treating ailments with miniscule amounts of natural substances to trigger the body to heal itself and restore balance. My background is in homeopathy, so throughout this book I have added some common homeopathic remedies that may be useful for treating minor ailments.

SUPPLEMENTS

Plants contain a plentiful supply of vitamins and minerals, often within an intricate and complex combination of biologically active chemicals. Nowadays these vitamins and minerals have become available as supplements, and it is perfectly possible to just 'pop a pill' to boost our diet with these essential compounds.

Indeed, the manufacture and sale of supplements is now a huge industry, so large that the new name

'nutraceauticals' has been coined for this sector, covering anything from diet pills to muscle-building potions. With so much money at stake, it is no wonder that we are bombarded with information on how these supplements will solve all our health problems; the fans of supplements also argue that the soil in which our food is grown has now become so denuded that we need them to supplement missing nutrients.

However supplements are expensive, and sometimes it is difficult for the body to digest, use and assimilate all the vitamins and minerals in them. The human body has evolved over thousands of years to use the plants around us for nutrition, while supplements have been around for less than a hundred years. Whether these modern alternatives are capable of replicating the vast diversity of the hundreds of phytochemicals, and the intricate balancing act these chemicals play within the plant, is still not clear.

I am not against taking some supplements at certain times of the year, or for certain conditions if recommended by a nutritionist, but in general I prefer to have fun making my own good health from what nature has to offer. It's easy, so why don't you give it a go, too?

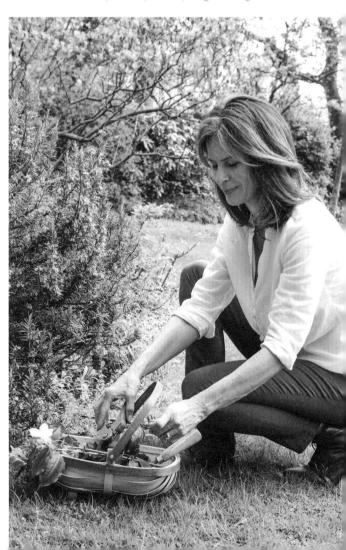

Techniques

There are many different ways that we can use the plants that grow all around us. Below I have suggested some of the methods you can use at home to harness the natural goodness of plants and enhance your health and wellbeing.

EXTRACTING THE GOODNESS FROM PLANTS

To make any recipe in this book you can use either dried or fresh plants. Drying plants is a useful method to keep those plants available to use in your recipes all year round (see Harvesting plants). Dried plants are more concentrated than fresh plants, so in any recipe less dried plants are needed.

To extract the goodness from a plant, you can either:

- Eat it raw: for example in salads, although this is only safe for some plants.
- Eat it cooked: for example in soups or jams, again only good for some plants.
- Soak it in alcohol or vinegar: so the plant's goodness can be absorbed by the liquid to create a tincture or vinegar, which you can then use internally or externally depending on the plant used.
- Soak it in hot or boiling water: so the plant's goodness can enter the water to create an infusion or decoction, which you can either drink or use in recipes for your skin, depending on the plant; alternatively, you can add the plant to a hot bath.
- Steep it in oil: to create an infused oil, which you can then use directly on your skin or in a balm.
- Apply it directly to your skin: as a compress or a poultice, again only a suitable method to use for some plants.

TINCTURES

Make a tincture with any part of the plant you choose: put it in a jar, cover it with strong 40 per cent proof vodka and then let it soak for at least two weeks (see Plantain tincture). The alcohol extracts the beneficial properties of the plant and acts as a preservative; if you don't like the idea of using alcohol, you can substitute it with vinegar (see Vinegars). Tinctures last a long time – on average three to four years – and they can be used either externally, or internally for some plants.

VINEGARS

Similarly to the action of alcohol in a tincture, vinegar is able to extract a plant's goodness. To make a plant vinegar, it is best to gently cook the plant in the liquid for a few hours. Although a vinegar is used like a tincture, it will not last as long – only up to a year.

DECOCTIONS

Decoctions are easy to make, using just water. Boil the plant in water for between 15 to 20 minutes so that all the goodness from the plant is extracted into the water. Once boiled, drain and throw away the plant and use the liquid either externally, or internally for some plants. The best parts of the plant to use for making decoctions are the 'tough' ones: the roots, woody stems, bark, seeds and berries. As decoctions are water-based, bacteria grows in them so they don't last as long as tinctures and vinegars: either use them straight away or add a preservative, such as sugar or citric acid. Decoctions are the base for many syrups and jellies, and are also useful for some skincare recipes.

INFUSIONS AND TEAS

Infusions are a simple, direct way to use many plants, just like making a pot or mug of tea. Place the leaves, flowers or soft stems of suitable plants in a mug or teapot and pour boiling water over them; after a few minutes the liquid can be used. Depending on the plant used to make the infusion, they can be drunk, inhaled or used externally as a wash or gel. Like decoctions, their water content means that they need to be used immediately.

INFUSED OILS

An infused (or macerated) oil is produced by adding a plant to a base oil, so that the oil takes on some of the qualities of that plant. There are two methods you can use to make infused oil. The first method involves covering the plant with oil then leaving it to seep in to it for two weeks, shaking occasionally and topping up with oil if needed, then finally draining to capture the oil (see Infused calendula oil). The second method involves gently cooking the plant in the base oil for several hours then draining to capture the oil (see Winter body scrub). When I make an infused oil I use sunflower oil as the base: it is generally found in kitchen cupboards, and it has a pleasant, light quality with no heavy smell or colour. Infused oils can be used directly on your skin or added to balms and other skincare recipes. Depending on the oil used, they can last for up to six months before the oil turns rancid.

COMPRESSES AND POULTICES

Both of these enable you to use the goodness of plants externally on your body, for example to treat a sprain, a sore shoulder, or even a cold. Make a compress by soaking a piece of cotton or muslin in the plant tincture or infusion, or by wrapping the plant inside the material. A poultice is similar to a compress, but the plant is used directly on the skin, held in place with a bandage. For example, a well known poultice is a cabbage leaf placed inside a bra to reduce the discomfort of swollen breasts during breastfeeding.

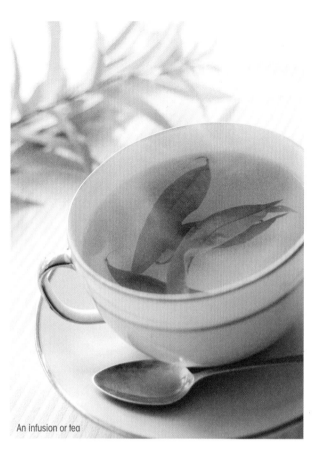
An infusion or tea

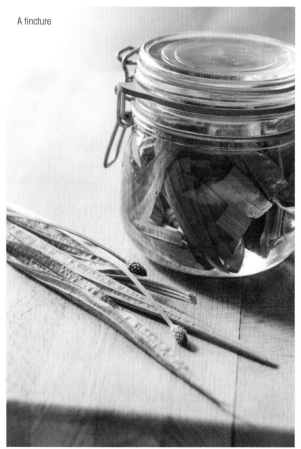
A tincture

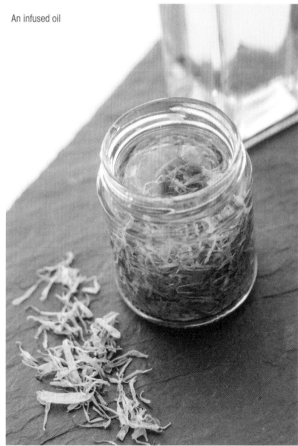
An infused oil

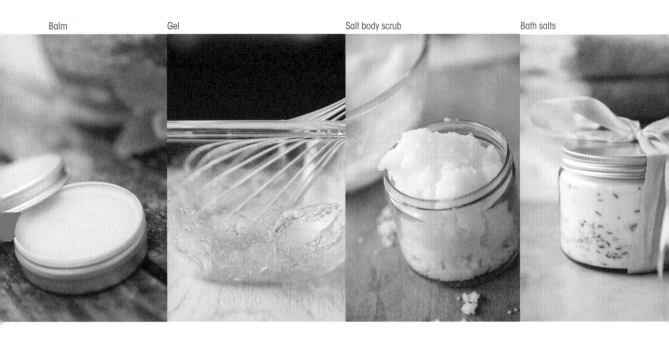

Balm   Gel   Salt body scrub   Bath salts

USING THE GOODNESS OF PLANTS

We have looked at techniques for extracting the goodness from plants by making tinctures, vinegars, decoctions, infusions and teas, infused oils, compresses and poultices. Now it is time to put these to use by looking at what we can make to enjoy the health benefits of this natural plant goodness.

BALMS

A balm is a completely oil-based product, with no water in it at all. It has a firm consistency, and is good for nourishing dry skin and lips. Balms are made from a combination of a wax (such as beeswax), a butter (such as cocoa butter or shea butter) and an oil (such as castor oil or olive oil).

Depending on the additional goodies you introduce in the form of tinctures and infused oils, balms can be used to treat different parts of the body. For example, if you add calendula oil, your balm will be soothing and healing; whereas if you use apricot kernel oil, your balm will be great for dry cuticles.

Balms are surprisingly easy to make: simply place your ingredients in a pan, gently melt, then pour into a pot (see Mint lip balm). Balms contain no water, which means that bacteria can't live in them so there is no need to add preservatives. However they still don't last forever, as the oils and butters in them do turn rancid after a while; depending on the oil you use, they will last from six months to a year.

OINTMENTS

These are essentially balms with a more runny consistency to make them easier to use for covering larger areas of your body. To make them follow a basic balm recipe, simply adding more oil (which is runny) and less beeswax (which is hard).

GELS

A gel has a jelly-like consistency, and turning water-based preparations like infusions or decoctions into gels is a useful way to make them thicker so they stay on your skin. To make a gel from an infusion or decoction, simply add a thickening agent, such as vegetable gelatine or xanthum gum. If you want your gel to last, you will need to use a tincture instead of an infusion for its alcohol content, which acts as a preservative, or add a preservative to the preparation.

TONERS

Toners can be a great addition to your skincare routine: used after cleansing and before moisturizing they will tone and refresh, often acting as astringents to help tighten pores. Toners can be as simple as flower water: for example, spritz rose water onto your skin to refresh it. Glycerine is used as a toner base, it is a sweet clear liquid that can act as a moisturizer and it is also found in cough and throat preparations. Add this to your infusions or tinctures to make them a little thicker, so you can apply them as toners to your skin with cotton wool.

HAIR RINSES

The goodness of plants can be used to treat various conditions of the hair and scalp (see Nettle and lavender hair rinse). Use an infusion or decoction as a final rinse to spray over your hair, or to massage into your scalp. Alternatively, add a couple of teaspoons of one of your homemade vinegars or tinctures to water and use in this way too. Rinses are great to enhance your hair's health.

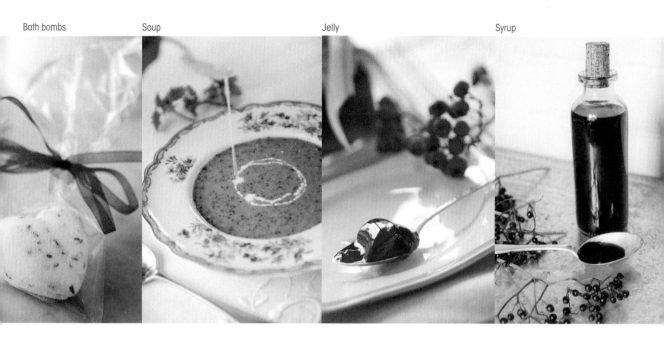

Bath bombs   Soup   Jelly   Syrup

BATH TIME

There are many ways to enjoy and benefit from the goodness of plants in the bath, and most are very simple. The easiest is to make a **bath soak**, by simply adding a handful of the appropriate plant parts to the bath water, or to make a **bath bag** by tying the plant in a bag of muslin and positioning under the hot running water (see Soothing chamomile bath soak). Or **bath salts** are super easy to make by mixing the essential oil or your choice with fine sea salt (see Relaxing lavender bath salts).

You can become more creative by making your own **bath bombs**: mix the plant of your choice with sunflower oil, bicarbonate of soda (baking soda) and citric acid, then set this mixture in moulds and leave to dry before using (see Lavender bath bomb). A **body scrub** is great for invigorating the skin and is made by mixing an infused oil with sea salt (see Winter body scrub). To make a **footbath**, heat a handful of plant leaves with water, simmer and cool then soak the feet (see Lavender footbath).

MOUTHWASHES AND GARGLES

Some plants have properties that help with oral hygiene, such as mint and clove, while others have antibacterial and antiviral properties that help with sore throats, like rosemary and garlic. This makes these plants great for cleansing and medicating the mouth and throat; simply prepare a decoction or infusion of the plant of your choice then rinse the mouth or gargle with it.

SYRUPS AND CORDIALS

Use your water-based preparations of edible plants to make syrups and cordials with water and sugar, adding citric acid as an additional preservative (although sugar does a good job of this if enough is used). In the context of this book the difference between a syrup and a cordial is really only one of name: you tend to use a syrup neat, either by taking a teaspoon daily, or pouring it over yogurt or ice cream (see Elderberry syrup); while you dilute a cordial to make a longer drink (see Elderflower cordial).

JAMS AND JELLIES

These are both delicious ways to consume the natural goodness of your herbs, fruit and berries. Like syrups and cordials, they are water and sugar-based, but the difference is you boil the jelly or jam mixture hard so it reaches a setting point of 104°C/220°F. For jelly you strain out the fruit or plant so you are left with a beautiful crystal clear jelly (see Rowan jelly), and for jam you leave this in (see Blackberry and apple jam).

SOUPS AND SALADS

Depending on the plant you've picked, you may have the option to eat it raw: I like adding some plant parts such as marigold petals or new dandelion leaves to salads, and adding herbs is always a delicious option. Other edible plants may need cooking, like nettles: the cooking takes out the sting, yet you still get the mineral and vitamin benefits. Making these into a soup provides an easy, nutritious and tasty meal (see Nettle and sorrel soup).

Basic Kit

I have tried to keep this book as easy to use as possible, so for most recipes all you will need is the plant you have gathered and your kitchen kit. However for some recipes you will need to source some specialized ingredients; once you have seen how easy it is to use these in your products, you will not regret buying them.

ESSENTIAL OILS

These are the natural, volatile oils contained within a plant that give the plants their fragrance: for mint these are found in the leaves, for roses they are found in the petals, for frankincense in the resin, and for ginger in the root. These oils are extracted through a complex process and this is why you cannot make these oils yourself, so you will need to buy them from a good health store.

Essential oils are highly concentrated and very strong, and are used as part of health and beauty treatments to bring the properties of that plant to the product. You can add a few drops of these to balms, ointments and other recipes found in this book. Essential oils must never be used neat on your body, as many can sting the skin or eyes. In addition, certain essential oils must never be used in pregnancy.

Having some essential oils readily available around the home is always useful, and some good ones to start off with include eucalyptus for colds, tea tree for spots, and lavender for relaxation.

BOTTLES AND JARS

Bottles and jars are used throughout this book for storing jams, jellies, syrups and many other health and beauty treatments. To ensure I always have a ready stock available for use in my own recipes, I collect all sorts of bottles and jars over the year, never knowing which size or shape will come in useful. In general I use glass bottles and jars where possible, as some plastics may leak into the product you make. Indeed, never use plastic for any hot products such as jams, or for any tinctures (with alcohol) or vinegars.

It is important that you thoroughly clean your bottles and jars before use. To do this, first soak them in hot soapy water to remove the labels. You may need to use a little white spirit to remove the glue, which will need washing off with soapy water. After washing, sterilize the containers to ensure they are completely free from bacteria. To do this you have two options: either pop them in the dishwasher so they are thoroughly washed and the heat from the drying programme sterilizes them; or wash them thoroughly in hot soapy water then put them in the oven on a medium heat (not too hot or the glass will crack) to warm and dry.

MUSLIN

Muslin is a lightweight cotton cloth that is ideal to use for lining a sieve for fine draining, as well as for making into parcels of plants for bath soaks. I suggest you purchase a large piece to keep in your kitchen drawer and use when needed; you can always wash it and re-use it.

WAX DISCS

If you are making jellies and jams keep a good supply of wax discs to put on the jars wax side down while the contents are still hot. These create an additional seal to further aid the preservation process.

LABELS AND RIBBONS

Adding a label to your preparations is crucial so you know what they are and when you made them. I love anything beautifully presented, and it doesn't take much to add your own touch to these labels with motifs or notes. If you are making a gift, a beautiful ribbon will add a final flourish.

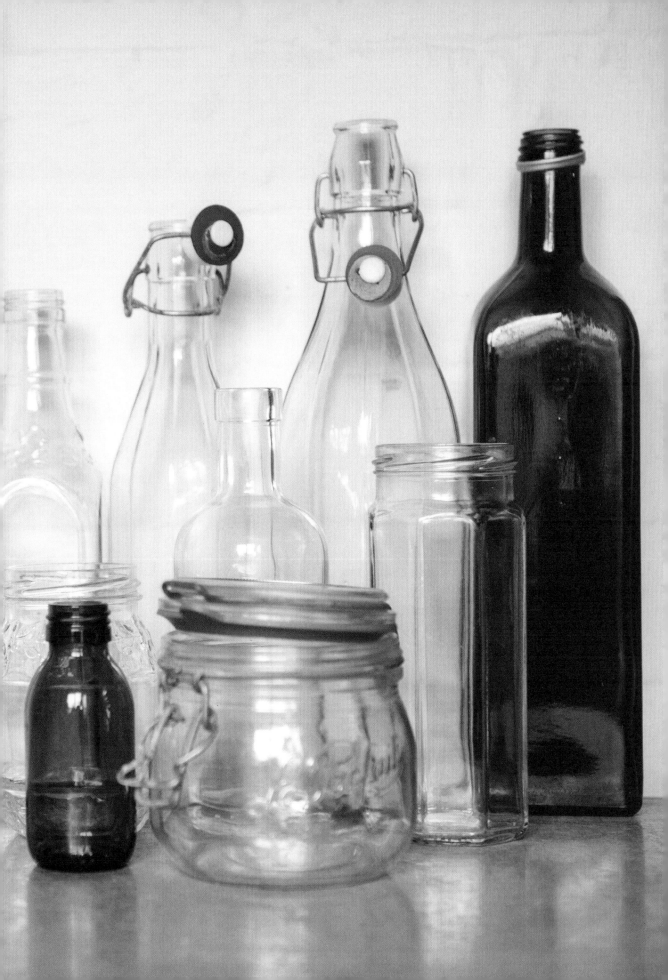

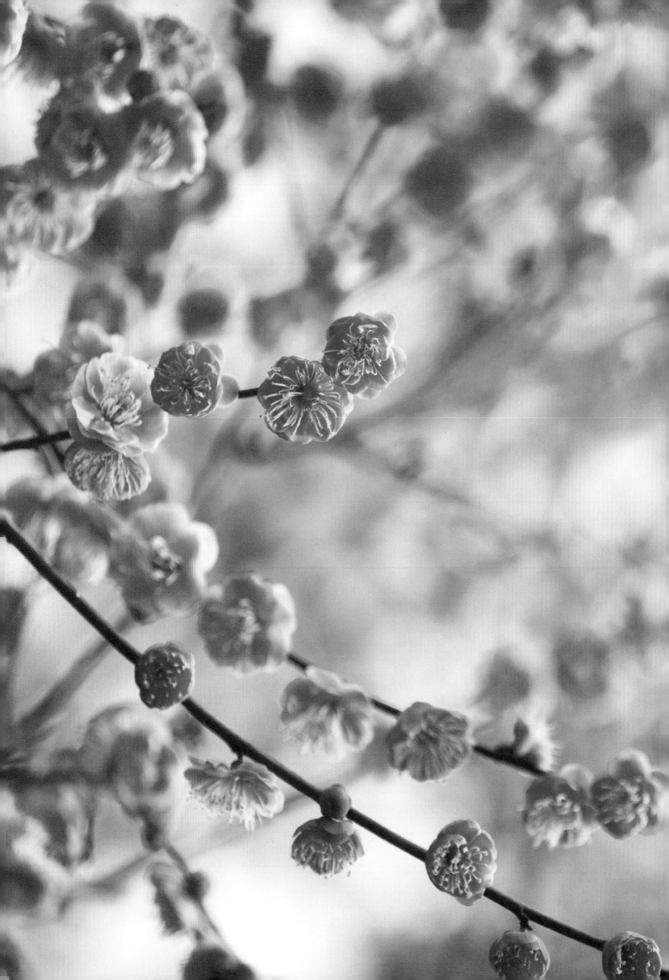

spring

As the days slowly lengthen, nature tentatively returns to life, as green shoots start pushing through the gradually warming soil and buds unfurl on bare branches. After a long cold winter, Mother Nature's pharmacy is waking up.

By late spring, it's as if nature has hit the fast-forward button – before you know it there are so many plants bursting with life, and fresh vibrant leaves – packed full of nutrients – are ready for picking.

Look out for the young leaves of dandelions and birch trees, which are both good for nutritious nibbles. And harvest the beautiful elderflower to create your very own delicious cordial.

Contents:

plantain: not the nuisance you think it is
dandelion: nothing goes to waste
common nettle: super soup and hair care
pucker up for st valentine's day: lip-smacking chocolate lip gloss
soil: more than it appears to be
beasties and beauties: a little about garden critters

horsetail: full of skin boosting silica
borage: essential in many ways
woodland wonders: two little plants to look out for
elderflower: no need to buy cordial again
bees: save the bees and all their goodness
yarrow: a natural wound wonder
hay fever: some natural ideas for relief

Plantain

Plantago Lanceolata

These so-called 'weeds' are the scourge of many a garden lover's lawn – but before you destroy them, think again. Plantain – or ribwort – is packed full of goodness, are great anti-inflammatories and antioxidants, and are packed with vitamins and minerals galore.

In my garden for stings, I use plantain in much the same way as dock leaves. So when I've been stung by a nettle, I simply rub my skin with either a crushed dock leaf or a crushed plantain leaf to help ease the pain. For general use, add a few handfuls of the leaves to make a calming and soothing bath for itchy, dry skin.

For cuts, plantain is good at drawing out any infection from a wound. This works best if you place the crushed underside of the leaves – the side with the ribs – on the affected area. Furthermore, if you are prone to hay fever these are the leaves to use for making a tea to help ease the inflammatory symptoms, as the plant will help to soothe the mucus membranes and also acts as an antihistamine.

plantain tincture

This is a standard tincture recipe that you can adapt for use with any plants. Always ensure the leaves are from an area that you know has not been sprayed with weed killer. Pure, strong vodka is the best alcohol to use for this tincture, but if you don't want to use alcohol, use vinegar instead.

what you need

- 1 jam jar
- Dried or fresh leaves to fill the jar
- Pure vodka to cover the leaves

1. Pick a couple of handfuls of leaves, shake them out to remove any bugs, and put them in a clean jar.

2. Pour alcohol (pure vodka is best) over the leaves, making sure they are completely covered with the liquid – if the leaves are exposed to the air they will rot.

3. Leave the mixture in the jar for two weeks, shaking occasionally.

4. After two weeks, drain and throw away the leaves, retaining the liquid as your tincture. This will last for two years.

5. If you don't want to use alcohol you can use vinegar, though you will need to cook the plantain leaves in the vinegar for two hours. The vinegar-based tincture will last for six months instead.

Sof SAYS... My daughter loves playing 'fencing soldiers' with plantain stems: each player picks a strong looking stalk and then tries to lob off the seedhead of their opponents with strategically placed, lethal blows. This is not as easy as it sounds!

recipe

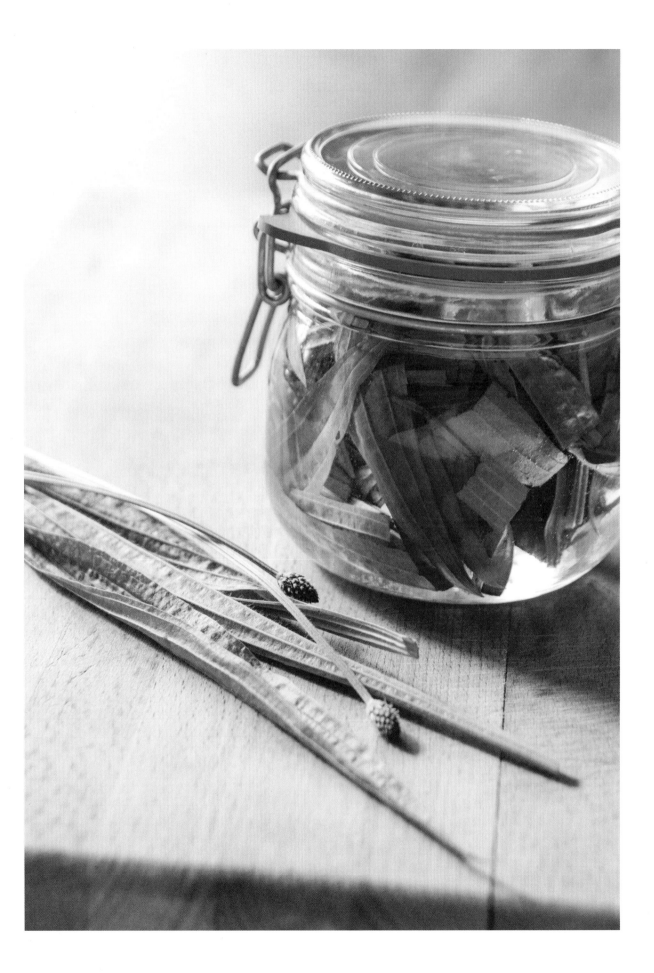

Dandelion

Taraxacum officinale

This cheerful little Spring flower is often taken for granted or treated as a weed to be eliminated. Yet think again, as every part of it can be used for your health.

LEAVES
The leaves are packed full of vitamin A, iron and potassium, and are great to drink as a cleansing tea.

ROOTS
The roots are full of tannins (naturally bitter components), and can be dried to use as a coffee substitute.

FLOWER
The flower can be fermented for dandelion wine, or used to make a soothing dandelion oil.

The dandelion is popular as a 'detox' herb, and is often used for kidney and liver concerns and to assist with water retention due to its diuretic qualities. In addition it is gentle on our stores of potassium, which other diuretics often leach out of the body. The bitter compounds found in the leaves aid digestion and the production of bile. Brew a tea from fresh or dried leaves, which will make an ideal after-meal drink to assist digestion, and will also act as a mild laxative.

The dandelion leaves have high levels of vitamin A and antibacterial properties, and this means they can help wounds and inhibit the growth of certain bacteria. This makes dandelion leaves a good skin tonic, either taken internally as a hot tea or applied directly to the skin as cooled tea. You can also add peppermint leaves, nettle leaves and fennel seeds to your dandelion tea to create a super powered skin cleansing tea.

For relaxation, the flowers can be used in a bath to help soothe aching joints and muscles: just put a handful in a square of muslin, tie up the parcel and leave it under the hot tap while you run your bath. Or try making an oil with the flowers that you can rub on any muscular aches and pains (see Pot marigold).

Joy SAYS...

Young dandelion leaves are a delicious – slightly bitter – addition to salads. The flowers, too, can be eaten in salads or fried in batter.

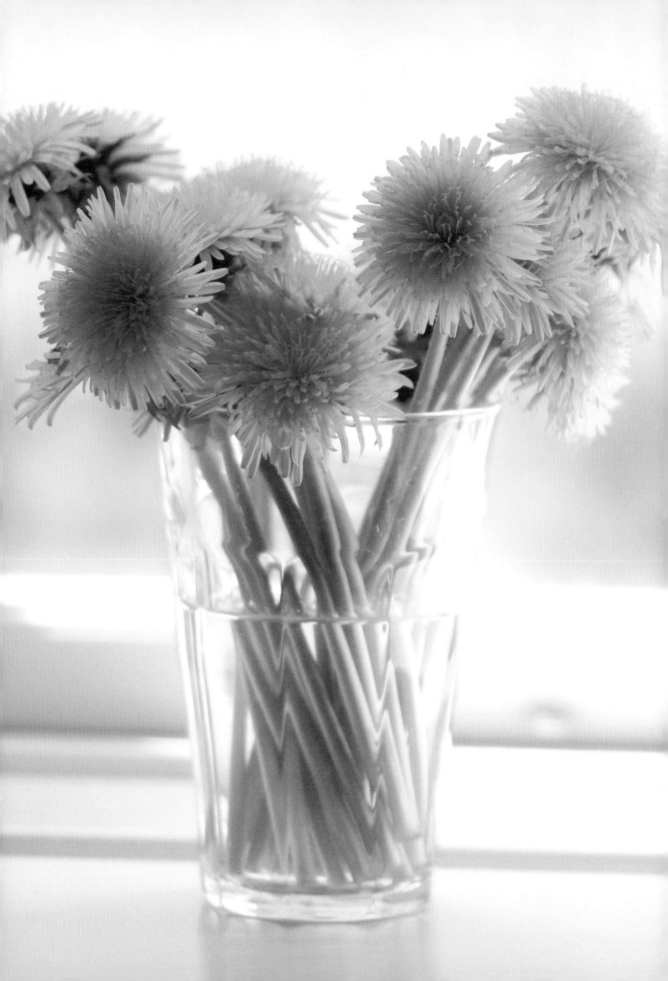

Common Nettle

Urtica dioica/Urticia urens

In a corner of my garden I have a flourishing nettle patch. Not only does this make easy gardening and provide a home to many moths and butterflies but, best of all, it provides me with a wonderful source of spring goodness.

Use young nettle leaves to make a great post-winter tonic, which is ideal for boosting our vitamin and mineral levels just when we need them most. The nettle's high iron levels make it good for anaemia and it also contains vitamin C, which makes it easier for us to absorb the iron.

nettle and sorrel soup

This is one of my favourite spring dishes, as it is tasty and nutritious; with its bright green colour it provides a real pick-me-up, heralding new beginnings. The sorrel gives the soup a delicious tart lemon sharpness and the nettle really does taste of minerals. A note: nettle leaves should always be picked with rubber gloves to avoid nasty stings, and only pick the top four or five young leaves.

what you need

- Approximately 20 nettle heads
- 1 handful of wild or common sorrel
- Water to cover the leaves
- 1 finely sliced potato
- 1 sliced onion
- 1 litre (1¾ pints) vegetable stock
- Salt and pepper
- Cream to finish
- Pan

1. Shake out any bugs from the nettle and sorrel leaves and put them in a pan, just covering the leaves with water.

2. Add the potato to provide the soup with thickness, and then add the onion for flavour. Simmer for 10 minutes.

3. Add the vegetable stock and cook your mixture for a further 10 minutes.

4. Let the soup cool a little before liquidizing, then season with salt and pepper to taste.

5. You can serve this either warm or cold; for a finishing touch, add a swirl of cream just before serving.

 Sof SAYS... You can dry the nettle leaves for use later in the year.

recipe

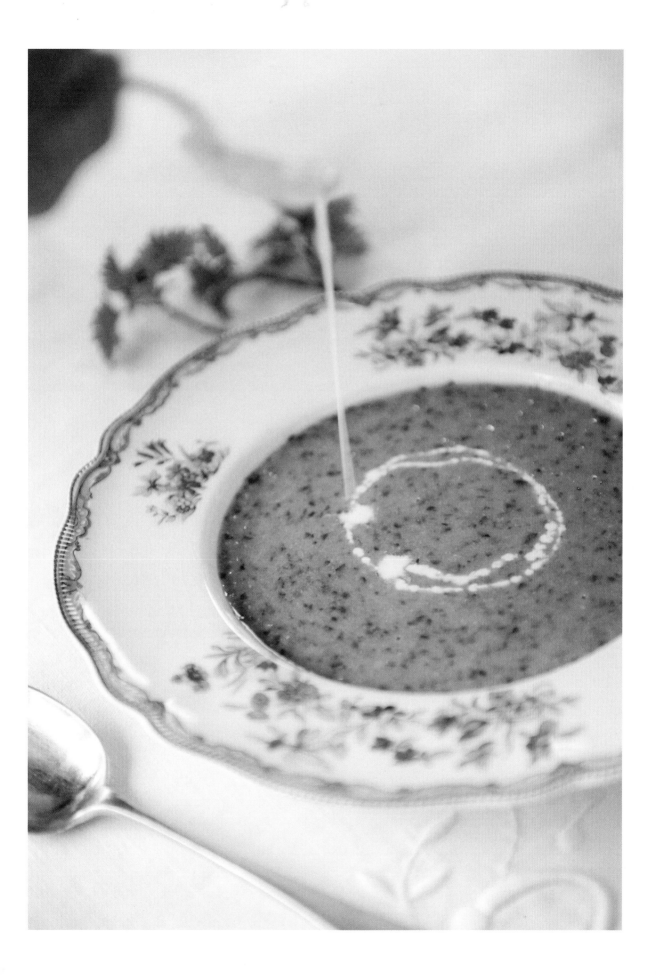

MORE USES FOR THE COMMON NETTLE

Not only are the leaves full of vitamins and minerals, but they also contain anti-inflammatories and natural painkillers that can help the pain and swelling of arthritis and rheumatism. Make a cup of nettle tea to assist this ailment, using fresh or dried leaves.

Even though nettles sting, nettle tea can help soothe hay fever types symptoms, due to its natural antihistamines. It is also used for cleansing oily skin and soothing sensitive skin, and may help with eczema due to its anti-inflammatory elements. Homeopaths use *urtica urens* for itchy skin, and it makes a great addition to a soothing balm combined with marigold and lavender. It is also said that the nettle root can help with enlarged prostate symptoms.

NETTLE AND LAVENDER HAIR RINSE

Nettles are said to stimulate hair growth. I am not sure if this is true, but the nettle certainly makes my hair feel softer, and look fuller and shinier. It is also good for dandruff and an oily scalp, as it increases blood circulation to the scalp area.

In fact, you will see nettle used in many natural hair care products, and you can harness its properties for yourself by making a nettle tincture (see Plantain). The tincture will keep for two years, so it's worth taking the time and trouble to make.

Use after shampooing. Mix two tablespoons of your tincture in a cup of water, add five drops of lavender essential oil to create a nice smell (nice, but not crucial) and spray over your hair, massaging into your scalp. There is no need to rinse this off.

When you make your nettle tincture, you could try adding some different leaves for additional benefits, as follows:

- For blonde hair you want to lighten a little more, add rosemary, chamomile or yarrow.
- For dark hair you want to keep dark, add sage.
- To reduce the impact of grey hair, add betony.
- For oily hair, add yarrow.
- To stimulate your scalp and for possible hair growth, try rosemary.
- For dandruff and a poor scalp condition, add rosemary.
- To stimulate hair growth, improve scalp condition, and to give your hair a shine, use young new birch tree leaves. These are better if used as a decoction (boiled in water), as the goodness is more easily released this way.
- To strengthen your hair, add horsetail – better if used in a decoction (boiled in water).

Add horsetail or birch leaves to any hair lotion you make, as they are full of saponins that will help open the pores of the scalp so the goodness of the nettles and the other plants can penetrate more easily.

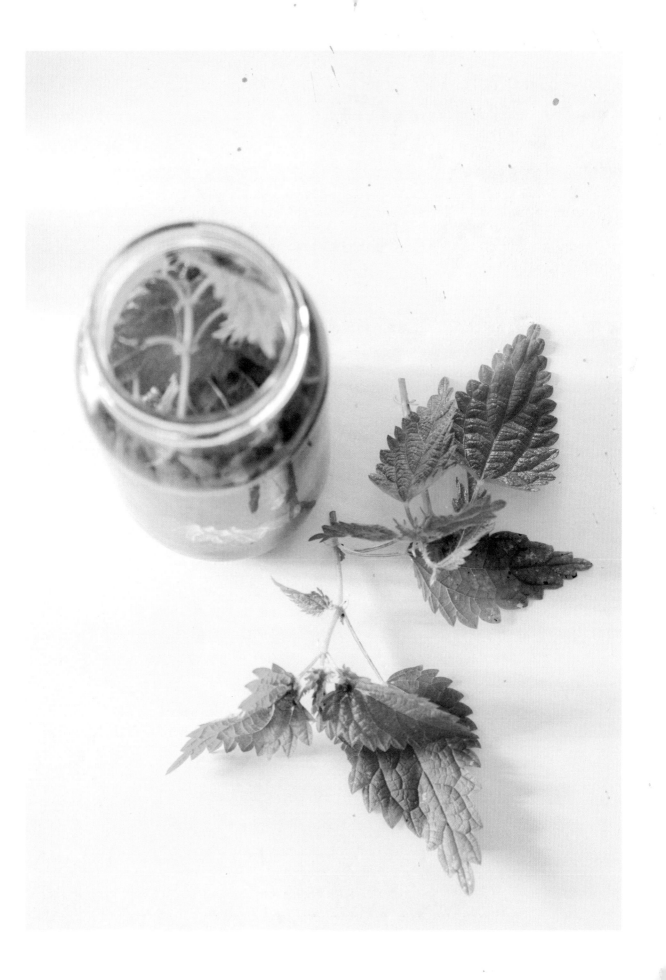

Pucker Up for St Valentine's Day

Luscious lips for St Valentine's Day is a must. Even if you've not got someone special in your life right now, just having smooth, well nourished lips can't be a bad thing. This is particularly important in the cold depths of winter when harsh, drying winds and cold weather mean lips need just that little extra care and attention.

chocolate lip gloss

This lip gloss recipe uses dark chocolate, which is reputed to contain a small amount of phenylethylamine, a chemical that mimics the hormone your body produces during sex. So not only will your lips feel gorgeous, but if you lick it off you'll feel fantastic too! The chocolate gives the lips a subtle, slightly darker sheen than clear lip balm; the castor oil gives them a gloss for super shiny lips; the cocoa butter is nourishing; while the beeswax protects the lips and gives the balm a good, firm density.

what you need

- 25ml (1fl oz) castor oil (or sunflower oil will do)
- 7g (¼oz) beeswax
- 12g (½oz) cocoa butter or shea butter
- 4g (⅛oz) dark chocolate (70 per cent cocoa solids works well)
- Small pan, with a lip if possible
- Small, clean glass pot with lid that will hold approximately 50ml (2fl oz)
- Kitchen paper (paper towels) for wiping up any excess balm mix

1. Put the castor or sunflower oil, beeswax, cocoa or shea butter, and chocolate in the small pan and gently heat until all the ingredients have melted. It is very important to do this gently and slowly; do not simmer at any point.

2. Once these ingredients have all melted, stir the mixture well.

3. Then pour it out into your pot, put the lid on, and leave to cool and harden for 30 minutes. A note: if you spill any of the mixture, use kitchen paper to wipe it up. Do not pour it down the sink, as beeswax can block the pipes as it hardens.

4. Once it has cooled, label your lip balm and enjoy your nourishing and moisturizing lip gloss.

5. As your lip balm is natural, made without any petroleum, it is more susceptible to changes in temperature. If it gets too hard, just put it in your pocket to warm it up a little; if it gets too runny, pop it in the fridge to harden up again.

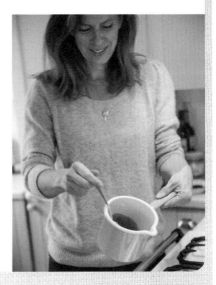

recipe

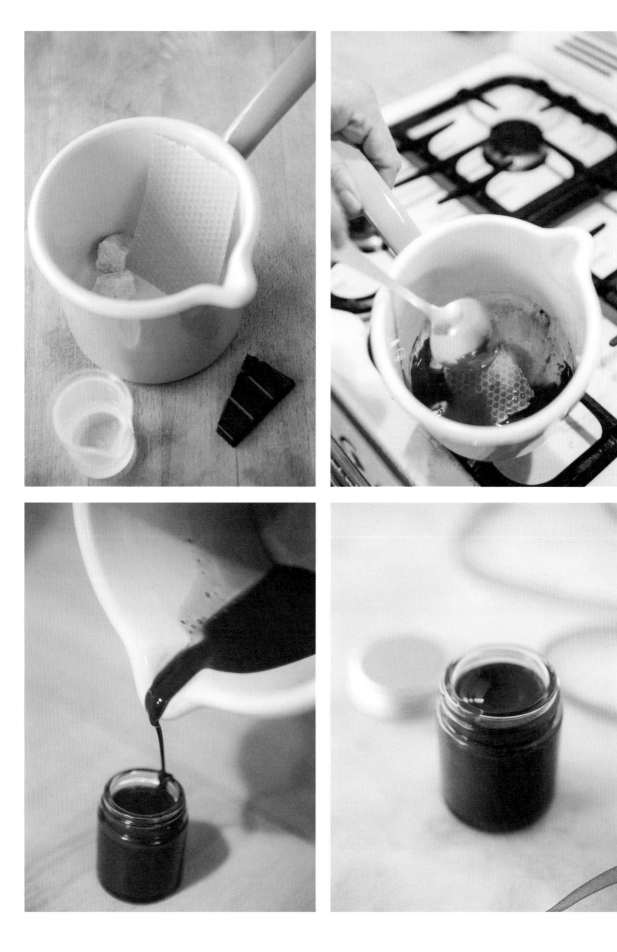

Soil

Soil itself is a wonderfully complex mix of billions of microbes, bacteria and nutrients. It's simple really: soil feeds the plants and we eat the plants, so a good soil is essential. A great way to garner all the natural goodness from the soil is to eat wild plants or 'weeds' that have often come from areas untouched by fertilizers and weed killers. The plants will break down each year and feed the soil in a natural cycle, a process that in turn feeds the plant we eat. To make the most of the goodness on offer, seek and collect wild plants – a process known as foraging – whenever you can. While doing this, make sure that you're not picking from contaminated wasteland or by a busy road, and also that you know what you're looking for.

Foraging is one way to avoid eating the mass-produced vegetables from today's new large-scale industrial farms, where the plants are grown on mineral wool and water with fertilizer added, a system known as hydroponic. I find this somewhat alarming if you are under the illusion that you are getting all your nutrients from these vegetables; how can this system replicate the complexities of 'real' soil? If foraging is not for you and nor is growing your own, then buy from your local farm shop, market or greengrocer so you can ask where the vegetables come from. Organic horticulture aims to produce healthy, good quality food in an ecologically responsible way, thus minimizing damage to the environment and wildlife.

Each country has its own organization for recognizing the provenance of food. In the UK the Soil Association has strict standards, so look out for their mark. In France the Ecocert system of organic certification labelling is very well respected. In America this is the Rodale Institute or the Organic Consumers Association. Most good organizations believe in the connection between soil, food, the health of people and the health of the planet.

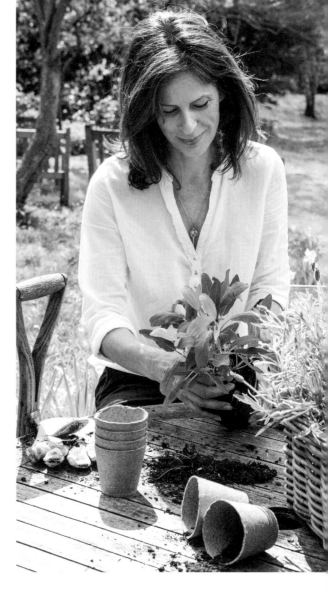

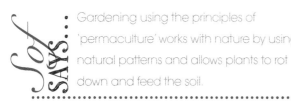

Sof SAYS... Gardening using the principles of 'permaculture' works with nature by using natural patterns and allows plants to rot down and feed the soil.

Beasties and Beauties

I can't write a book about healthy plants and not mention some of the little beasties that help or hinder these plants, from slugs and caterpillars to bees and butterflies, they all play an important role.

SLUGS AND SNAILS

These much-maligned creatures are normally seen as the foe of gardeners and plants alike. Indeed, I agree that there are few things more disheartening for a hardworking gardener than to find favourite hostas, lupins or lettuces munched to nothing almost overnight. But there's no need to reach for the slug pellets. Slugs are beloved of hedgehogs, and song thrushes love snails, so don't poison them; just keep them away from your favourite plants. To do this, I recommend using crushed eggshells.

Over the winter months we collect and crush all our eggshells, so by Spring we have a good bag full to scatter around the new shoots of slug prone plants. So far, so good – we've managed to stave off these little critters. Furthermore, slugs can be used for your 'health': I have a friend who is something of a white witch who swears that if you put a slug on a stubborn wart, it will shrivel and disappear. However I was unable to try this on my daughter's wart – she point blank refused to put a slug on her skin, and I don't blame her!

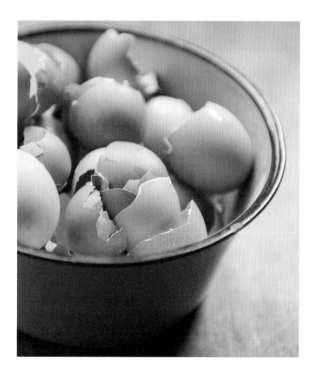

BEES AND BUTTERFLIES

For the past seven years we've been gardening without pesticides or herbicides. This was not an intentional decision; more to do with not quite getting to grips with the garden, so letting nature run its course made sense – that is, once I'd wrestled the slug pellets out of my husband's grasp. Although now I wouldn't garden any other way and in terms of wildlife, this policy is starting to pay off: our garden is now host to many pollinating bees (see Bees), native ladybirds that eat aphids, and beautiful butterflies, many of which rely on weeds such as nettles to hang their cocoons from.

'Butterflying', as Winston Churchill called it, gave him great pleasure: he remarked at the age of only six

'that I am never at a loss of what to do in the country, as I will be butterflying all day'. He was to continue his love of 'butterflying' right through his Prime Ministerial days during the Second World War. I find this insight into how a great head of state switched off from running the country fascinating, and a reminder that the beauty of nature can be a source of great happiness.

If you garden, don't be over zealous in your tidying. Some butterflies need to overwinter on plants, and bees need nooks and crannies in which to 'nest'.

Horsetail

Equisetum arvense

Horsetail, commonly known as bottlebrush, is incredibly strong and has even been known to push up through stone patios, breaking them apart. In actual fact, it contains one of the highest amounts of silica of all known herbs. Silica or silicon is the second most abundant element on earth after oxygen and makes up a quarter of the earth's crust. Compounds of silicon are found in all natural waters and in many plants and animals, and it is vital for good skin, ligaments, tendons and bone function.

Horsetail can be used to help strengthen connective tissue and skin cells, and it is useful for psoriasis and eczema sufferers as it is thought to promote new skin cell production. Horsetail leaves can be used externally on the skin or taken internally, drunk as a tea. However take care: horsetail is also a diuretic increasing urination, thus long-term use is not recommended. You can also obtain a homeopathic remedy of silica, and this is wonderful for skin and nails.

horsetail conditioning nail ointment

Due to its high silica content any horsetail preparation is ideal for strengthening nails. Here I have combined it with apricot kernel oil, which is very hydrating for the skin around the nails and is therefore often found in cuticle care products. You can buy the horsetail tincture ready-made, or create your own from dried or fresh leaves (see Plantain tincture).

what you need

- 15g (½oz) beeswax
- 3 tsps (15ml) sunflower oil
- 70ml (2½fl oz) apricot kernel oil
- 20 drops of horsetail tincture
- Small pan
- Small pot, approximately 100ml size

1. Melt the beeswax and sunflower oil in a small pan very slowly on a very low heat; this process should take less than a minute.

2. Remove from the heat and add the apricot kernel oil.

3. Then add the horsetail tincture and stir it into the mixture well; the beeswax will help the oil to absorb the alcohol from the tincture.

4. Pour the ointment out into a small pot then rub it into your nails and cuticles nightly.

recipe

 Sof SAYS... Never pick your own horsetail unless you are absolutely certain of it, as there are many poisonous plants that look almost identical to it.

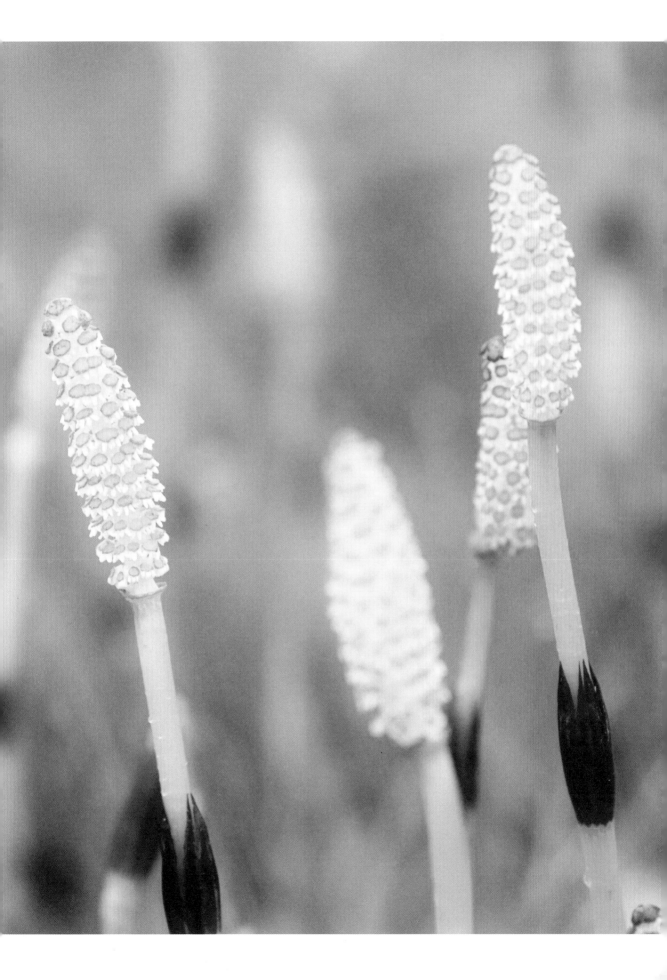

Borage

Borago officinalis

This pretty, spring plant is an early flowerer along with forget-me-nots, though borage is easier to spot as it is fairly hairy. Another name for borage is 'starflower' after its delicate flowers and it's from these flowers that come the seeds, which is what concerns us here. These seeds are packed full of a very special omega – gamma linolenic acid (GLA). This is a form of omega 6, and also occurs in the more well known evening primrose oil, as well as in small amounts in hemp and blackcurrant seed.

GLA is excellent for skin complaints such as eczema and scar treatment, and is also known to aid pre-menstrual complaints and joint swelling; simply rub borage oil into the skin on the affected area. Making your own oil from the seeds is not easy, so I would recommend buying borage oil from a herbal supply company. Borage oil doesn't smell great, so for external use I also add a few drops of lavender essential oil to improve the fragrance. Check with your health care provider before taking borage oil internally as it can react with some medicines, especially non-steroidal anti-inflammatory ones. In addition, long-term use of borage oil is not recommended, and neve for pregnant women.

ESSENTIAL FATTY ACIDS/OMEGAS

The GLA in borage oil is an essential fatty acid – or omega – and having fatty acids in our diet is good for us; the 'essential' in their name gives it away, as they are essential for normal health and growth. Modern diets are often devoid of essential fatty acids and are instead full of saturated fats, such as butter and lard, or hydrogenated fats, like margarine.

Essential fatty acids are vital for every cell in our body and they are particularly helpful for many skin complaints, arthritis, coronary heart disease, pre-menstrual tension and bone loss in menopausal women, in addition to healthy brain development in children.

Well known natural sources of essential fatty acids are fish oil and flaxseed (or linseed) oil, which is full of omega 3. When buying flaxseed oil, ensure it has not been exposed to heat, light or oxygen, as this causes it to go off, leaving you with a rancid oil bereft of all benefits. Once opened, it has a short shelf life of about two weeks.

Pour one tablespoon of flaxseed oil over your food just before you eat, as it has a delicious nutty taste. However don't cook with it, as the heat destroys any health benefits of the oil.

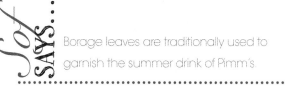 Borage leaves are traditionally used to garnish the summer drink of Pimm's.

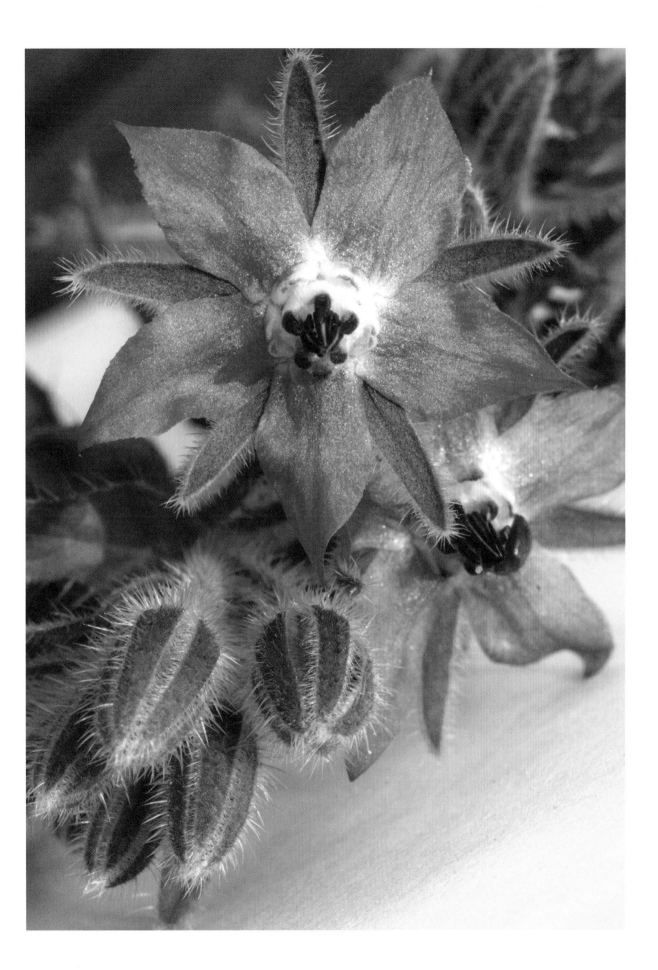

Woodland Wonders

As the days start to warm up, a woodland walk is a fantastic way to shrug off any Winter doldrums. Seeing spring bulbs like bluebells and daffodils will lift your spirits, but don't overlook these two small woodland wonders.

WOOD SORREL
Oxalis acetosella

Wood sorrel is very different from the more dock-like leaves of common sorrel (rumex). Wood sorrel is a small, delicate woodland plant, with tiny light green, clover-like leaves that have a habit of pointing upwards, like a pyramid. Wood sorrel has a delicate light lemon tang and can be added to salads – it's too tiny for soups. On the other hand, the large common sorrel with its strong tangy lemon flavour is great to cook with (see Nettle and sorrel soup) and is also incredibly easy to grow, coming back year after year; all you have to do is pick it.

SWEET WOODRUFF

Galium odoratum

This little woodland plant forms neat clumps about 15cm (6in) high, and has small white star-shaped flowers in late Spring. Despite its Latin name *gallium odoratum*, neither its flowers nor leaves smell of much -- until they're picked and start to dry. Aha! Now the name makes sense. The resulting sweet smell is wonderful: freshly mown hay with an underscent of marzipan.

The dried leaves retain this smell, so they are great to add to potpourris or make up fragrant bunches for linen cupboards. Alternatively, use them to brew a soothing tea that will help insomnia and anxiety. Traditionally, sweet woodruff was used to aid liver function and help with gallstones.

However be warned: too much of this little plant can induce dizziness and vomiting, owing to the very chemical that provides it with its sweet smell, coumarin.

Sof SAYS... Sweet woodruff was traditionally used to flavour May wines and beer.

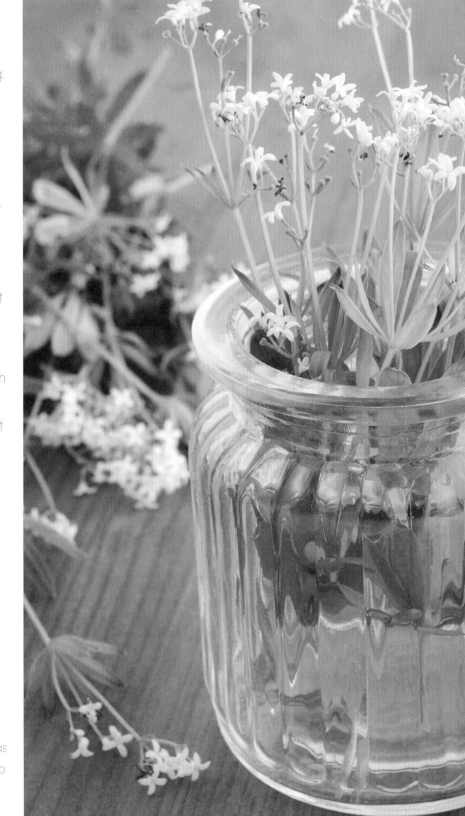

Elderflower

Sambucus nigra

For most of the year the common elder is almost unnoticeable, sprouting up on wasteland with the ease of the purple buddleia. Yet for a few weeks in late spring and again in autumn this large shrub comes into its own, with its bounteous array of uses.

The large, flat saucer-shaped white flowers of the elder are distinctive, and best picked when open but not starting to 'go over'. Their scent is wonderful and heady in spring, so try to capture this by using the flowers straight after picking.

The flowers, like the berries, are antiviral, so are good for treating spring coughs and colds. They are also a good decongestant, loosening catarrh and soothing irritated throats. It is easy to make a tea or a gargle with one or two flower heads to treat these ailments, adding sugar or honey according to your taste.

If you have oily congested skin, try making a steam facial with the flowers as they can help clense pores: just put four or five flower heads in a bowl of recently boiled water and hold your face over the steam, being careful not to burn yourself.

elderflower cordial

This is now a familiar sight on supermarket shelves, but it is very easy to make your own. You are aiming for a subtle balance of tartness and sweetness, without destroying the delicate elderflower flavour. The recipe provided here will last for several months, or you can freeze it.

what you need

- 60 elderflower heads
- 5 unwaxed lemons
- 3 litres (5¼ pints) water
- 2.5kg (5lb 8oz) caster (superfine) sugar
- 125g (4½oz) citric acid
- Sieve lined with muslin
- Large bowl
- Large pan
- Clean, sterilized bottles or jars

1. Shake out any bugs from the flowerheads and place them in the large bowl (or in several bowls).

2. Zest then slice the lemons and add to the flowers in the large bowl.

3. Now make a sugar syrup: fill a large pan with half the water and add all the sugar. Heat just until all the sugar is dissolved, stirring all the time. Do not burn!

4. Pour this sugar syrup over the flowers and lemons in the bowl then add the rest of the water.

5. Sprinkle over the citric acid and stir well.

6. Leave overnight so the elderflower flavour and goodness can seep out into the water.

7. In the morning, strain the mixture through a sieve lined with muslin. Push out as much liquid as you can; squeezing the muslin with your hands at the end is messy but satisfying.

8. Pour this liquid into clean, sterilized bottles or jam jars (see Bottles and jars).

9. You can use your cordial straight away – just dilute with water to taste.

 Sof says... Traditionally the flowers were used at summer weddings to bring luck and fertility. So when you next go to a wedding, scatter them freely instead of confetti!

recipe

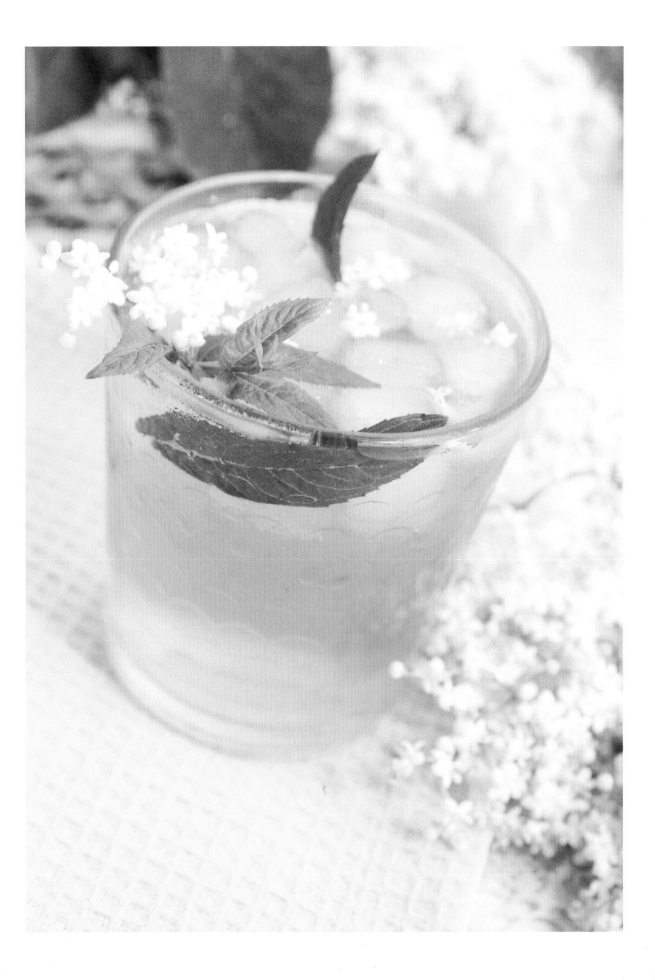

Bees

At last a sign of warmer days to come – the first bees. As they drowsily emerge from hiding you know the seasons are changing and summer is just around the corner. The survival of bees is important for many reasons; not just because they pollinate a huge number of our crops upon which we rely, but also because the produce of bees provide many health benefits.

HONEY

We all know how delicious and sweet bees honey is and what's more, it is packed full of goodness and health benefits. It will help to soothe sore throats and coughs, and eating a spoonful of honey from local bees is said to alleviate some types of hay fever. Honey contains antibacterial elements that are good for healing minor wounds; simply dab it carefully on the affected areas. Finally, honey is full of antioxidants, which means that it can nourish, replenish and revitalize your skin, and makes a wonderful addition to a skin scrub. Do note that honey is not suitable for infants under the age of one year due to certain natural bacteria contained within it.

BEESWAX

Beeswax is the wax substance secreted by bees to make honeycombs, and I use beeswax on a daily basis as one of the ingredients in the lip balms I make. There are many different grades of beeswax to choose from; ones used for candles are obviously not as good and pure as ones used in cosmetics, so choose carefully. Beeswax is widely available to purchase, but when doing so I do like to discover where the bees that are making a particular wax are from, and what they are feeding on, so always ask about this.

PROPOLIS

Propolis is a product made by bees to protect their hives from infection. They produce it by collecting resin from the buds, leaves and bark of trees and plants, then mixing it with beeswax and enzymes. It has been recognized for decades for its antiviral and antibacterial properties, as well as being antiseptic, anti-inflammatory and antioxidant. There are several propolis products on the market that range from syrups and throat sprays to lozenges. However be sure to use it with caution, as it can induce an allergic reaction.

HELPING THE HONEY BEE

The plight of the bee has been well publicized of late, but what can we do to help?

If you're a gardener you can:
- Grow the plants bees love: simple, single flowers are best, like foxgloves, comfrey and lupins, as well as many herbs, such as chives and sage.
- Reduce the use of weed killers; especially neonicotinoid pesticides, as these are linked to the decline of bees and banned in many countries.
- Keep areas of the garden 'untidy' with nooks and crannies for some bees to live in.

Even if you are not a gardener, you can:
- Buy organic foods, as neonicotinoid pesticides are not used in their production.
- Buy cosmetics from companies with bees and their survival at the centre of their philosophies, such as Melvita from France, or Comvita from New Zealand.
- Support the ban of neonicotinoid pesticides in your country – some countries like France and Germany have already done this – or support a campaign to encourage less intensive single crop farming.

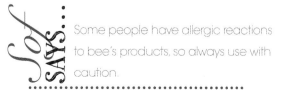

Some people have allergic reactions to bee's products, so always use with caution.

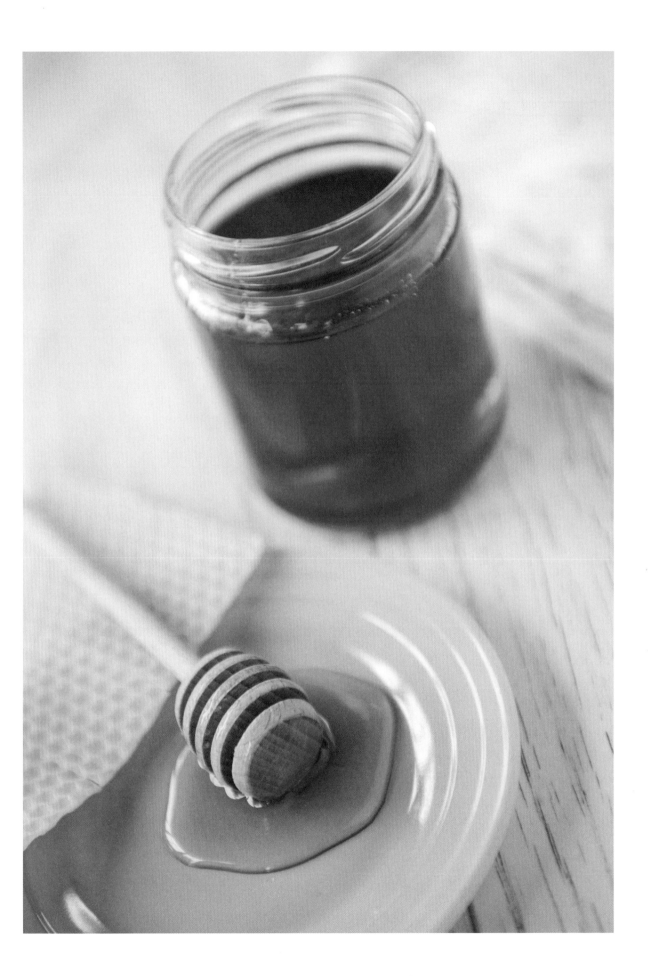

Yarrow

Achillea millefolium

I first discovered yarrow as a child. Bewitched by Cicely Mary Barker's *Flower Fairy* books, I was envious at the beautiful blonde Yarrow Fairy who appeared to be identical to my big sister, while I resembled something more akin to the small, chubby brunette Clover Fairy. So I always look on the plant with love, even when it pops up where it shouldn't be, as it can be quite invasive. But gardeners relax; if you see it in your prized borders, folklore says the ground is blessed. Foragers will find yarrow in hedges and unfertilized fields.

Yarrow can be confused with other plants that also have white flowers – for example, the poisonous hemlock – so be sure you have picked the right plant. Look carefully for its distinct feathery leaves, and 'if in doubt leave it out' of your foraging basket.

USES FOR YARROW

For generations yarrow has been known as 'woundwort' and 'staunchweed', which gives us a clue to one of its uses. Indeed it used to be packed into wounds to stem the blood flow, owing to its haemostatic (blood stopping) properties. To help alleviate nosebleeds, simply crush up some leaves and plug them into the bleeding nostril. Due to its effects on the blood, drink yarrow as a tea to help regulate the blood flow of a period if it is too scanty or too heavy. A word of caution around its effect on the blood: do not use when pregnant, and never use yarrow on a long-term basis.

With antiseptic, anti-inflammatory, astringent and drying properties, yarrow is a good plant to use externally on varicose veins and haemorrhoids. These are the same properties that make yarrow good for skincare, as it will help to strengthen skin tone, and alleviate eczema and oily skin problems. To use yarrow on the skin, make a tincture of the flowers then either add to a toner or ointment. Yarrow relaxes skin pores, thus allowing sweating in the early stages of fever, which can be helpful to reduce the body temperature. Andy Hamilton, a British forager who specializes in drinks, recommends making and drinking yarrow, peppermint and elderflower tea at the first sign of a cold.

When using yarrow, be aware that most of the active ingredients are to be found in the flowers. These contain salicylic acid, which has pain relief properties and is the main ingredient of aspirin. Leaves are also used, but they are not as strong as the flowers.

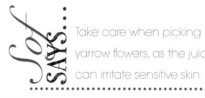 So SAYS... Take care when picking yarrow flowers, as the juice can irritate sensitive skin.

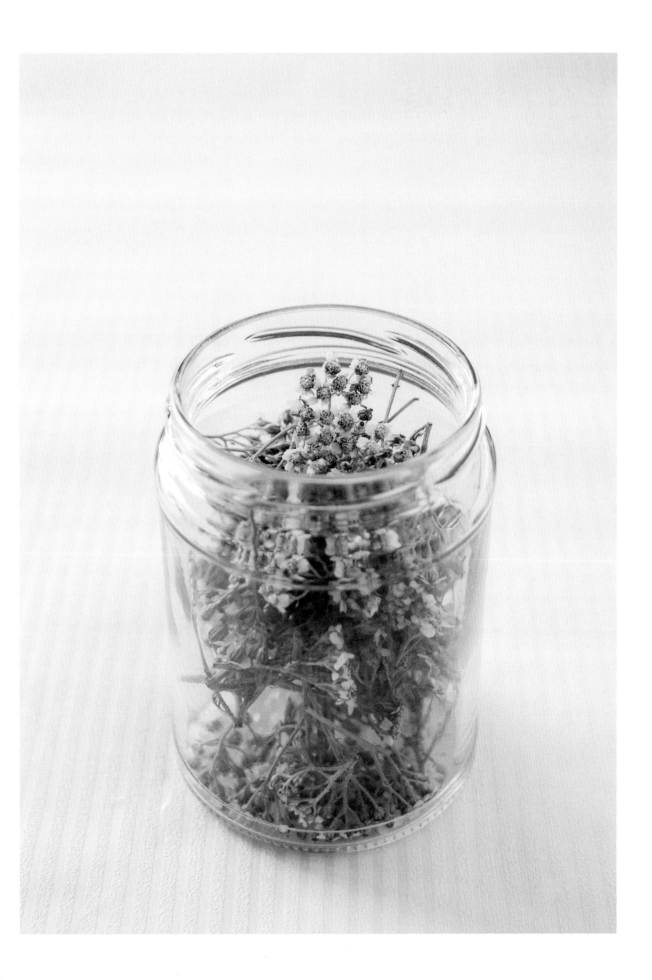

Hay Fever

Late spring is the time of year when hay fever strikes, and depending on your particular allergies, your life can become a misery for the next few months as different plants emit their pollen. Essentially, if you are allergic to something your body treats that substance like a foreign body, attacking it as part of its immune response with histamine. An overzealous histamine response can cause uncomfortable effects, thus the use of an antihistamine to subdue these. Allergies often run in families; as a child I was highly allergic to dust amongst other things for which I was given an antihistamine pill called triludan, which is now banned. I am therefore always on the look out for natural remedies that may help me; below are some ideas that may help you do the same.

RELIEF THROUGH DIET

One idea to help with hayfever is to try to build up your own natural antihistamine levels and reduce other factors that may increase histamine. You can help your body to do this by avoiding foods that contain a high level of histamine. Nature creates histamine in food and drink as bacteria decays, so avoid aged red wine, aged cheese and smoked food; basically, fresher food contains less histamine.

Fresh fruit and vegetables are crucial for effective histamine metabolism, not only for their vitamin content but also because some contain quercetin, which is thought to be anti-inflammatory and possibly antihistamine. Good natural sources of **quercetin** are red onions, kale, watercress, legumes, apples and some berries. A tea made from the leaves of plantain can also help relieve some histamine symptoms (see Plantain).

Sot SAYS... If you have a serious allergic reaction, you must seek immediate medical help.

EUPHRASIA/EYEBRIGHT

Unless you live in a mountainous region, you will probably not come across this pretty little plant in the wild, although it can also grow well in pots. The leaves, stems and flowers of this plant are used for herbal remedies, and it is best collected in midsummer when it is in full flower. Many people find euphrasia helpful for hay fever symptoms, especially any eye-related ones. One of the reasons it is thought to work is that it contains **aucubin**, a glycoside with antihistamine and anti-inflammatory properties.

Herbalists have been using euphrasia to treat eye conditions for centuries, and now it is commonly used to make a tincture that is taken internally; diluted in a few drops of water, to ease certain eye symptoms. For example, it may help with itchy eyelids, acrid burning tears, oozing pus, sticky eyes, a painful gritty feeling as if sand is in your eye, and even intolerance to bright lights; it's also worth trying for conjunctivitis or any catarrhal eye infection. Homeopaths use it for the same eye-related conditions.

RELIEF THROUGH HOMEOPATHY

Depending on your particular hay fever symptoms, certain homeopathic remedies may help to relieve some of them. Some of the stalwarts in the homeopathic pharmacopeia for hay fever are available in pill form, so ask your pharmacist about the following:

- **Allium cepa**, otherwise known as the common red onion. Think of how you are when you cut an onion: streaming eyes and runny nose, when the amount of liquid produced seems large and bland rather than itchy. These are the symptoms this homeopathic remedy helps.
- **Euphrasia** is the Latin name for eyebright and is useful for any type of eye symptom, including either itchy or runny eyes (see Euphrasia/Eyebright).
- **Sabadilla** may help to alleviate spasms of sneezing.
- **Wyethia** may help an itchy pallet, mouth and nose, when the itching is driving you mad.
- **Arundo** is for a tickly nose and ears.
- **Nux vomica** is good for treating blocked up noses, headaches and an irritable mood.

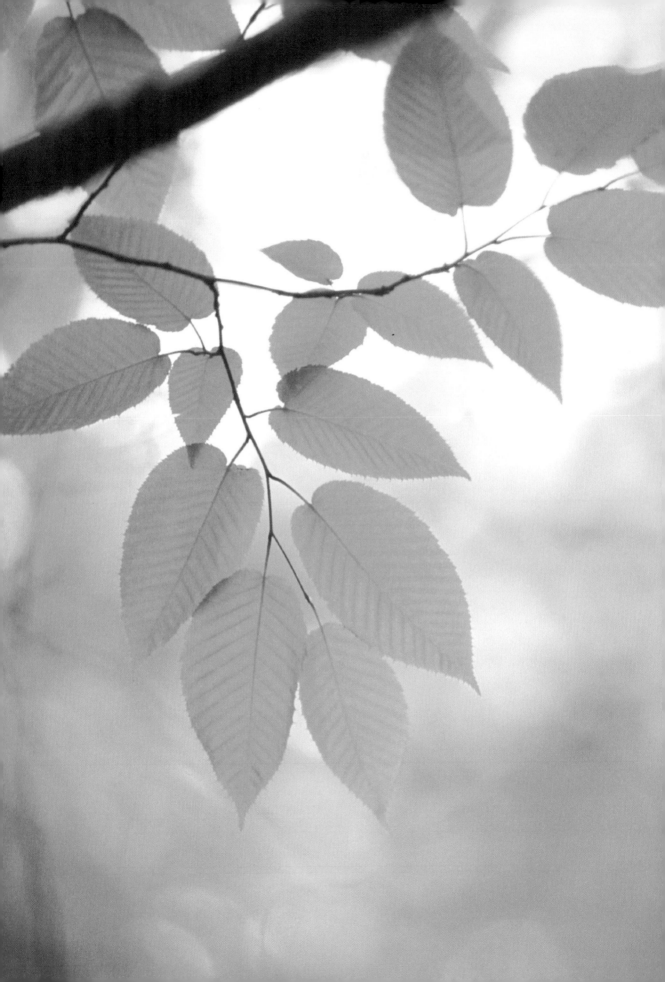

summer

At this time of year nature is in full spate, with flowers abundant and all looking rich, lush and ripe for the picking. I become ridiculously excited about what summer promises, rushing around looking for flowers just blooming, previously unseen butterflies, and new little plants. Yet the best moments are just stopping and enjoying it all.

Contents:

pot marigold: the skin-soothing queen
chamomile: calming bath soak
travel: a queasy-free trip and your own first aid kit
rose: a pretty teatime treat and much more
comfrey: the Florence Nightingale of plants

oils: not just for eating
lavender: bath bomb bonanza
lady's mantle: skin toner tannins
mint: balm for fresh lips
harvesting plants: drying for use all year round

Pot Marigold

Calendula officinalis

This cheerful orange flower is commonly known as pot marigold, but it is its Latin name, calendula, that you will see in lists of ingredients on health and beauty products. As it is easy to grow, it is a must for any garden and also looks lovely grown in a large pot.

The pot marigold is my absolute number one plant remedy for skin complaints: it can help to speed up the healing process of minor rashes and grazes; it is soothing due to its anti-inflammatory properties; and it is a great remedy for dry flaky skin. Follow the recipe below to make an oil to treat these various skin complaints.

infused calendula oil

Making an oil from the flowers of the pot marigold is very easy, and the process allows the goodness from the petals to seep out into the oil, which you can then use. This will provide an excellent addition to any home remedy cupboard.

what you need

- 1 sterilized jam jar
- Fresh or dried petals to half fill the jar
- Bowl
- Sieve lined with muslin
- Sunflower oil to fill the jar

1. Half fill a jam jar with dried or fresh pot marigold petals.

2. Pour sunflower oil over the petals and fill up to the top of the jar, making sure all the petals are covered – this is important, because if the fresh petals are exposed to air they can become mouldy. Give the mixture of oil and leaves a good stir, making sure there are no bubbles left in.

3. Leave the jar in a warm spot – on a windowsill or in an airing cupboard – for two weeks. During this time check the petals are still covered in oil, and top up the oil if you need to. This process allows the natural goodness of the petals to seep in to the oil.

4. After two weeks, drain the contents of your jar through a sieve lined with muslin into a bowl. Squeeze out the muslin to extract all the goodness, keeping the oil then pouring it back into your jar for use. This will be a lovely rich orange colour and will last for six months.

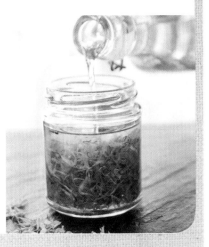

Sof SAYS...

You can eat pot marigold flowers; they look very pretty scattered over a salad.

recipe

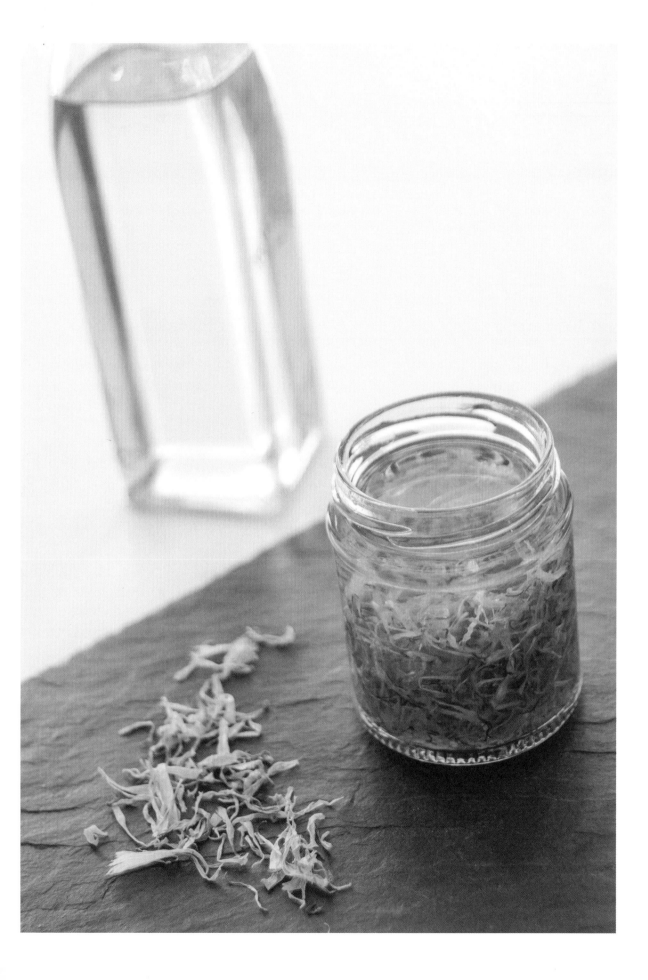

USES FOR INFUSED CALENDULA OIL

Your rich, orange calendula oil is wonderful to use neat on your skin, rubbed into dry rough areas; it is also useful for soothing sensitive, red and flaky patches of skin. As with all skin treatments, always carry out a sensitivity test first, as everyone's skin sensitivity varies. Your oil will make a great base for making a balm: simply add some beeswax to help solidify the oil and some cocoa butter for extra nourishment that will work well on winter lips (see Mint lip balm).

The skin soothing anti-inflammatory qualities of marigold petals can also be used in a bath: scatter a handful in a hot bath, or tie them in a square of muslin (less messy when you come to drain out the bath). These same qualities also calm and soothe digestive disorders; make a cup of marigold flower tea after eating to help alleviate digestive complaints. You can collect the fresh petals throughout the summer months and dry them as you go, to ensure you have a plentiful supply for the winter.

GROWING POT MARIGOLD

When choosing pot marigold plants or seedlings, don't get confused with the French marigold, marsh marigold or others members of the tagetes genus. To avoid confusion, look out for its specific Latin name, *calendula officinalis*, which is usually written in brackets somewhere on the pack. Pot marigold is a perennial, which means that it can come back year after year, but sometimes it won't survive a hard Winter. So it is best to only think of the plant lasting a year, but in that year it will put on a really great show, pushing out lots of flowers. Indeed if you cut the flowers, the plant will flower again and again. Flourishing in most soils, marigolds love a sunny spot and also grow well in a pot. They are rampant self-seeders, so if you have an area in your garden where you can just leave them to seed, they can return year after year.

 Sot says... A shortcut to making a muslin bath square is to simply cut the foot from an old pair of clean tights and fill it with pot marigold petals.

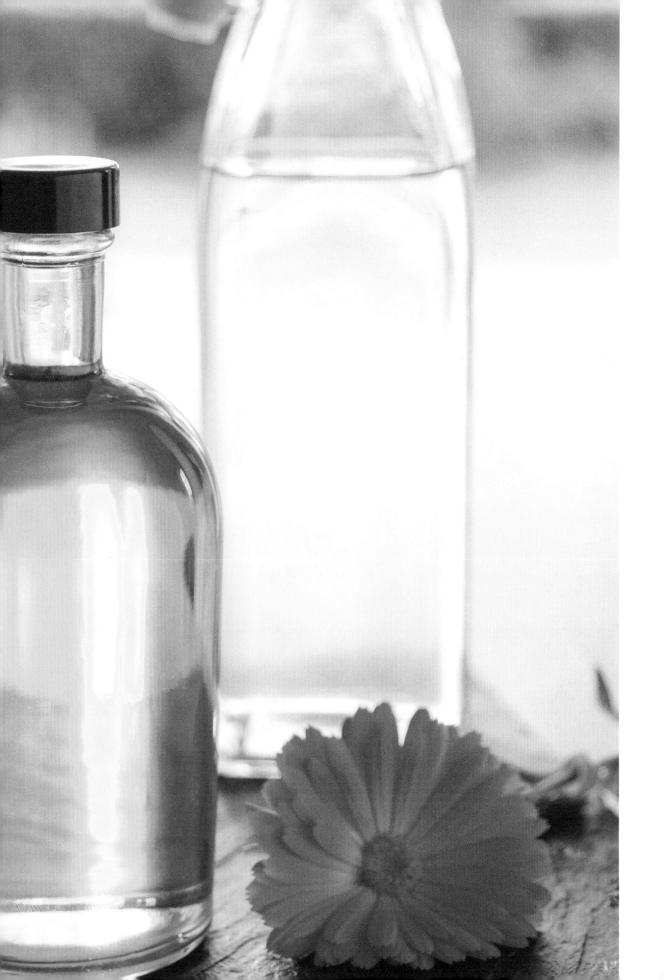

Chamomile

Matricaria recutita, chamaemelum nobile, chamaemelum treneague

My father once grew a small chamomile lawn; in the summer it was soft and springy to walk on and smelt heavenly, almost like apples. Garden lore says that if you place a chamomile plant next to a sickly plant it will recover.

Drunk as a tea, chamomile is one of my favourite all-round home remedies. Its relaxing, sedative properties are well known, hence its appearance in numerous bedtime teas; lifting the spirit and soothing the soul. In addition, it is a great aid to digestion as it has anti-inflammatory and antispasmodic properties relaxes the smooth muscles found in the gut.

Used externally, chamomile has an antibacterial effect on the skin and is often used to calm weeping eczema, haemorrhoids, varicose veins and mouth sores. I find an infusion of chamomile useful for minor conjunctivitis and eye discharges when there is no obvious cause. Just make sure you let the infusion cool before using, then dab onto the affected eye with cotton wool.

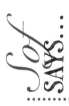 *Sof SAYS...* If you can't find dried chamomile flowers, try using the contents of a good quality organic chamomile tea bag instead.

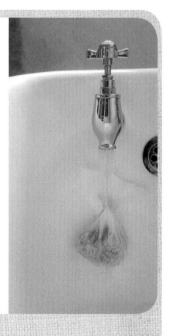

ramomile bath soak

Not only is chamomile soothing for your skin, but as you inhale the hot water vapours of chamomile in a bath you'll relax, and all unhelpful thoughts will slip away. The oats in this soak add a skin-softening element and also have a calming effect on dry itchy skin. The chamomile itself is calming and soothing, and will help any inflammations.

what you need

- 1 tbsp organic oats
- 2 tbsp dried chamomile flowers
- Square of muslin

1. Mix the oats and dried chamomile flowers together and place on a square of muslin.

2. Tie up the muslin and hang the parcel under the hot tap of the bath, letting all the goodness into the bath as the water runs.

3. Add cold water to suit your preferred bath temperature.

recipe

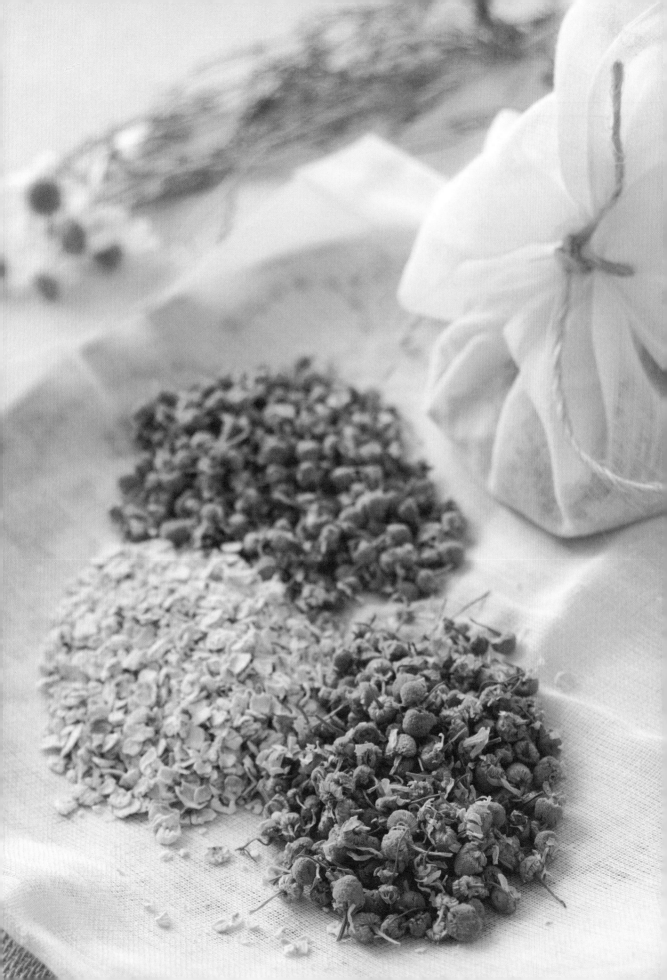

Travel

Summer is the time of year when vacations beckon, and with them comes the prospect of travels near and far.

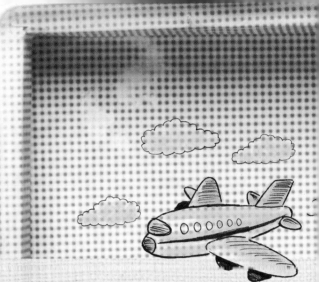

TRAVEL SICKNESS

Many people love travelling, but what if the very thought of travel and motion makes you feel queasy? Don't worry, as there are several alternative remedies to try to relieve the discomfort.

- **Acupressure bands** are elasticated wristbands with a small bead designed to apply pressure to the point on your wrist that relates to nausea in acupuncture. I find these bands even work for seasickness, and are available in children's sizes, too.

- **Ginger** in any form is good for nausea and sickness. Take it either as sweets to suck on; in biscuits, as tea, or freshly added to a homemade juice (see Ginger).

- **Ipecac** is a homeopathic remedy derived from the coffee plant family and is good for nausea, especially if vomiting doesn't relieve the symptoms

- **Homeopathic cocculus** is worth trying if dizziness accompanies nausea. It is also good for vertigo, so take some with you if you're planning a sightseeing trip up tall towers.

AIR TRAVEL

More often than not, travel involves a flight. If air travel makes you nervous, try the classic homeopathic 'fear remedy', aconite. Or try Rescue Remedy, which is a herbal flower essence that can be calming; traditionally this was sold in drops, and is now even available as a chewing gum.

If you are concerned about earache during air travel, I was given the following excellent tip by an airhostess when my daughter was screaming in agony as our flight was landing. Handing me two plastic cups with just an inch of hot wet kitchen paper (paper towels) at the bottom, she told me to hold these cups to my daughters' ears, taking care not to get any hot wet paper on her. The result was instant: somehow the heat, moisture and vacuum created affected the pressure in my daughter's ear and she stopped screaming at once – a relief for all!

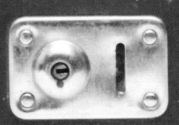

FIRST AID KIT FOR TRAVEL

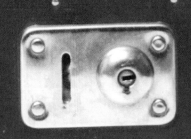

Packing for your travels is one thing, but the prospect of taking a huge medicine bag along with you to treat travel ailments can seem daunting. So here are my top five alternative must-haves for a vacation first aid kit – and they are all small items too:

- **Aloe vera gel or cream** is made from the leaves of the tropical aloe plant, and is great for soothing itchy hot sunburn or rashes from nettles or insect bites. If you don't have this to hand, I find that vinegar helps to soothe the tight heat of mild sunburn; gently dab it on with cotton wool, and don't worry – the smell evaporates quickly.

- **Arnica** is the one homeopathic remedy that many people have heard of. It is good for bumps and bruises, as well as unexpected trips wearing flip-flops!
- **Carbo veg** is vegetable charcoal in a homeopathic formula. I find it invaluable for tummy upsets of the gassy indigestion type, which often accompany trips to warmer climes as our digestion tries to adapt.

- **Citronella spray** is made from a grass-like tropical plant of the same family as lemon grass, and it keeps mosquitoes and midges at bay. There are several lotions available on the market, which have citronella mixed with other essential oils such as lavender and eucalyptus to stop the citronella becoming too overpowering. Never use an essential oil neat on skin because it's very strong and can sting; instead, always dilute it with a base oil.

- **Belladonna** is homeopathic deadly nightshade, but don't worry because it is so diluted that no molecules remain. This works wonders on sudden hot fevers and infections. Belladonna is also good for throbbing ear infections, which can appear quite suddenly from swimming and turn any subsequent flights into nightmares.

Rose

Rosa

Even on a dull summer's day, the soft scent of the blowsy rose by my backdoor
is enough to conjure up thoughts of the warm summer sun with bees buzzing,
when nothing is remotely urgent. So it is no surprise to learn that aromatherapists
use the essential oil from roses to calm stress-related conditions and to lift the
spirits. Roses have many uses in skincare, coming later, but first here is a childhood
favourite of mine.

crystallized rose petals

When I was a child, for my summer birthday my mother held a rose-themed party for me. Everything was
pink, and we ate rose petal sandwiches and crystallized rose petal cakes – it was heavenly! Make your
own crystallized rose petals by following this simple recipe; it is fun to make with children as the sugar
and egg white can get quite sticky.

what you need

- 1 handful of rose petals
- 1 egg white
- 1 small bowl of caster
  (superfine) sugar
- Small brush
- Greaseproof (wax) paper

1. Take a handful of your favourite rose petals, ensuring they have not been sprayed with anything harmful. The stronger the scent of these petals, the stronger their taste will be – although the flavour of roses is always very subtle. Scatter them on a plate, allowing time for any insects to hurry away.

2. Some roses have a strong white section where the petals attach to the flowerhead. These can sometimes be quite bitter to eat, so you can snip them out with a pair of scissors using a little triangle snip.

3. The next stage must be done petal by petal, which sounds laborious, but by enjoying the wonderful scent of the roses it can be incredibly relaxing. Lightly fork up one egg white then use it to gently cover both sides of your first petal with a brush. Dip both sides of the petal in caster sugar then place it on the greaseproof paper to dry. Repeat the process with the other petals.

4. Once all the petals are covered, you can use them immediately as decorations on cakes, or store them in an airtight container in the fridge for several days.

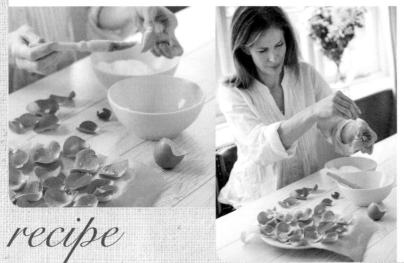

recipe

Sof SAYS... Put rose petals in a
sandwich sprinkled
with sugar for an easy
and pretty snack.

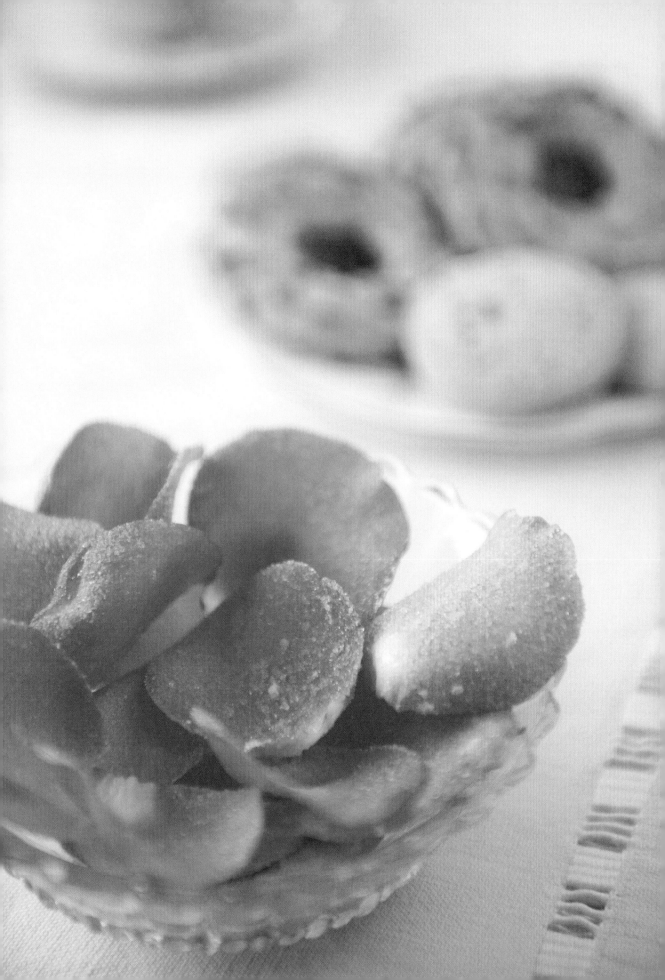

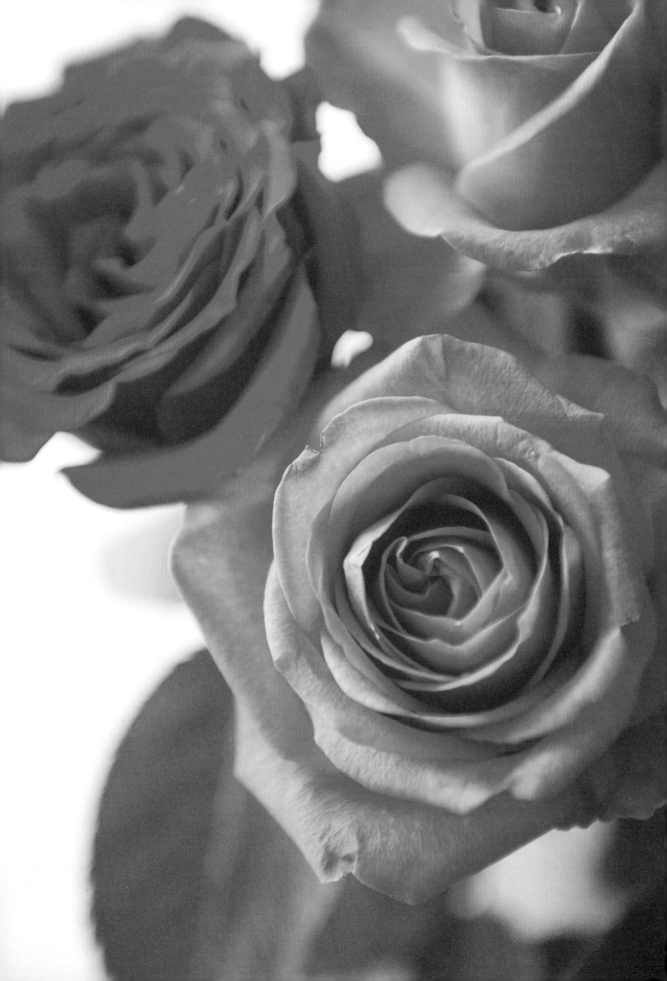

USES FOR ROSES

The scent of roses not only soothe emotions but it is these same oils that also soothe agitated skin conditions, and rose oil is one of the best essential oils for harmonizing and balancing the skin. Rose oil is particularly good for dry mature skin, and also has calming properties that will ease skin inflammations.

Another use for rose petals is in your bath to help cool and soothe sunburnt and itchy skin. Simply add a couple of handfuls of petals to the hot running water. If you are worried about blocking the drain by adding the petals directly to the bath water, wrap the petals in a square of muslin and hang this under the running tap instead (see Soothing chamomile bath soak).

It is easy to make your own infused rose oil that will provide you with a delicate oil to use in balms or directly on your skin. To do this, follow the recipe for calendula oil (see Infused calendula oil), simply replacing pot marigold petals with rose petals. This is an easy way to get the most out of roses, and much more cost effective than buying rose essential oil, which is one of the most expensive oils to buy.

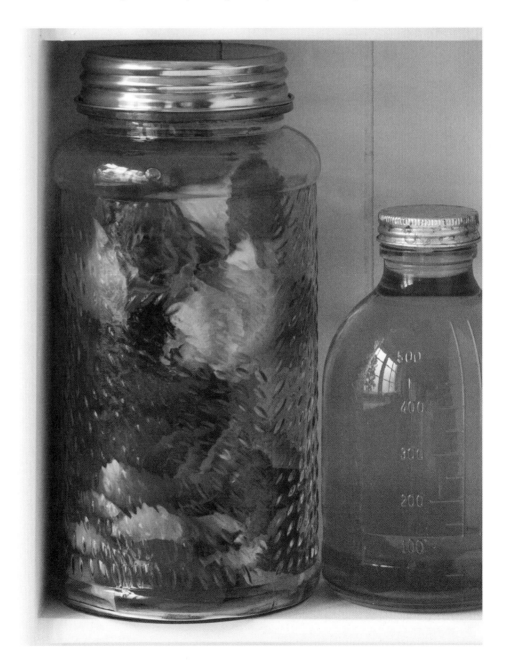

Comfrey

Symphytum officinale

Comfrey is well known to gardeners as it makes an excellent fertilizer for strong and robust plants; it is easy to grow, has a pretty flower, and comes back year after year. It has also been widely used in herbal medicine for years, but internal use of the root is now banned as prolonged use can cause liver damage; and internal use of the leaves can only be carried out under the advice of an experienced herbal practitioner, and in some countries this is not allowed either. Do not use comfrey if you are pregnant or breast feeding.

Comfrey has a high carbohydrate content, which if used externally is thought to soothe and rejuvenate the skin, and it also contains the phytochemical allantoin, which has properties that aid skin cell regeneration and encourages the growth of healthy cells. These qualities make comfrey useful for calming and soothing itchy skin, and for helping wounds or sores that won't heal, varicose veins, stubborn leg ulcers, gout and other inflammations. To treat these, try making and applying the root gel in the recipe below.

The traditional name of comfrey is 'knit bone' or 'bone set', and for years it has been used to do just that, helping to promote bone growth after damage. You will need to see a herbal practitioner if this is your concern. Homeopaths also use comfrey for this, under its Latin name symphytum.

comfrey root gel

Follow this recipe to prepare a light gel that will soothe dry, itchy skin and help regenerate any skin cell damage.

what you need

- 100g (3½oz) washed and peeled comfrey root
- 1 gelatine sachet or 1 tsp xanthum gum
- 1 litre (1¾ pints) water
- Pan
- Bowl
- Sieve
- Small, clean pot
- Optional: ½ tsp Preservative 12, used in the vegan food industry in Denmark

1. Peel the fresh comfrey root, chop it up and put it in the pan with the water.

2. Bring the water to the boil for five minutes then turn down the heat to a gentle simmer. Leave this to simmer for two hours to let the mucilage release, topping up the pan with extra water if needed.

3. After two hours you will see how glutinous the root has become due to its high mucilage content. Drain the contents of the pan through a sieve into a bowl and set the liquid aside to use for your gel.

4. To make the gel, sprinkle the xantham gum into the comfrey liquid, whisking it in well. Alternatively, use the comfrey liquid to make up the gelatine according to the packet instructions, stirring it well; only use half the amount of gelatine so you have a loose rather than firm jelly.

5. Add the preservative and leave to set. If you have not used preservative, your gel will last in the fridge for one week; with the preservative, it will last for a month.

recipe

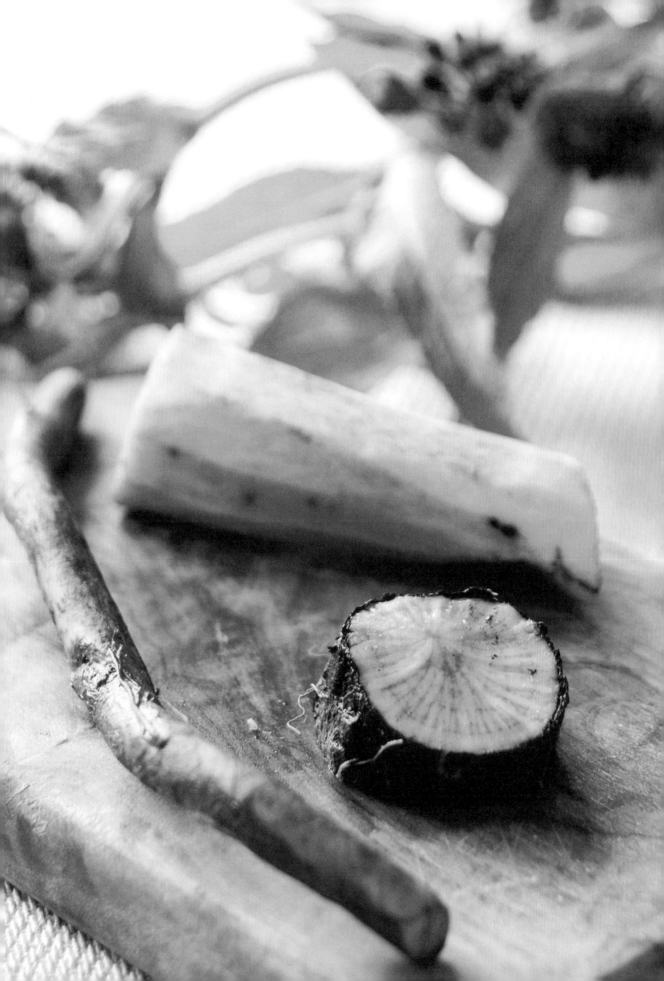

Oils

For me, an important part of summer days are the long lazy lunches with fresh salads, drizzled with generous helpings of virgin olive oil. Vegetable oils are great, not just to eat, but many are used in skincare products. In fact natural skincare relies heavily on different oils, butters and waxes, all offering something slightly different for the skin.

Most oils can penetrate the skin to some degree and as oils carry fat-soluble nutrients, the skin can benefit from them. All oils have their own characteristics – for example dry, light, heavy or fatty.

Extraction is the name of the process by which oil is obtained from nuts, fruits and seeds. This process can be as simple as a small oil press squeezing out the oil, but commercially it is now done on an industrial scale using several techniques. The following are a brief description of these, so you will know what to look out for:

- **Cold pressing** extracts the oil without heat and produces a fine high quality result – for example cold pressed virgin olive oil.
- **Hot pressing** applies heat, thus more oil can be extracted by using this method. For some oils, this method can compromise the quality of the product.
- **Refining** is a process that most oils undergo to some extent as a form of cleansing. Some oils also need refining to remove a bitter taste or overpowering smell, so it can be a necessary process.
- **Dry or light oils** seems an odd way to characterize oils, but certain ones are definitely less fatty and sticky on your skin than others. For example thistle and rose hip oils are dry, making them ideal for use on skin that is prone to large pores and oil secretion.
- **Fatty or heavy oils** tend to be the oils from the nut family – for example, macadamia oil and shea butter oil. They are great for moisturizing cracked dry skin on hands and feet, but don't use them on facial skin with enlarged pores.

BUTTERS AND WAXES

Butters are thicker than oils, penetrate deeper into the skin, and are useful to help maintain the skin's natural moisture; shea butter and cocoa butter are two well known examples. Waxes are absorbed very slowly into the skin, often forming a protective barrier from the elements. As the melting point of cocoa butter is 35°C (95°F), whereas beeswax is considerably higher at 63°C (145°F), waxes are often used in skin products so they maintain a firm consistency that won't melt easily.

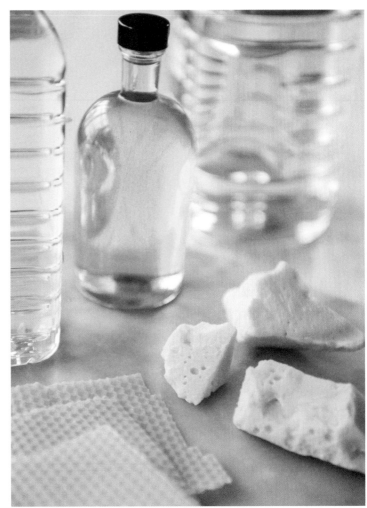

Sunflower oil, Bees wax, Calendula oil, Cocoa butter

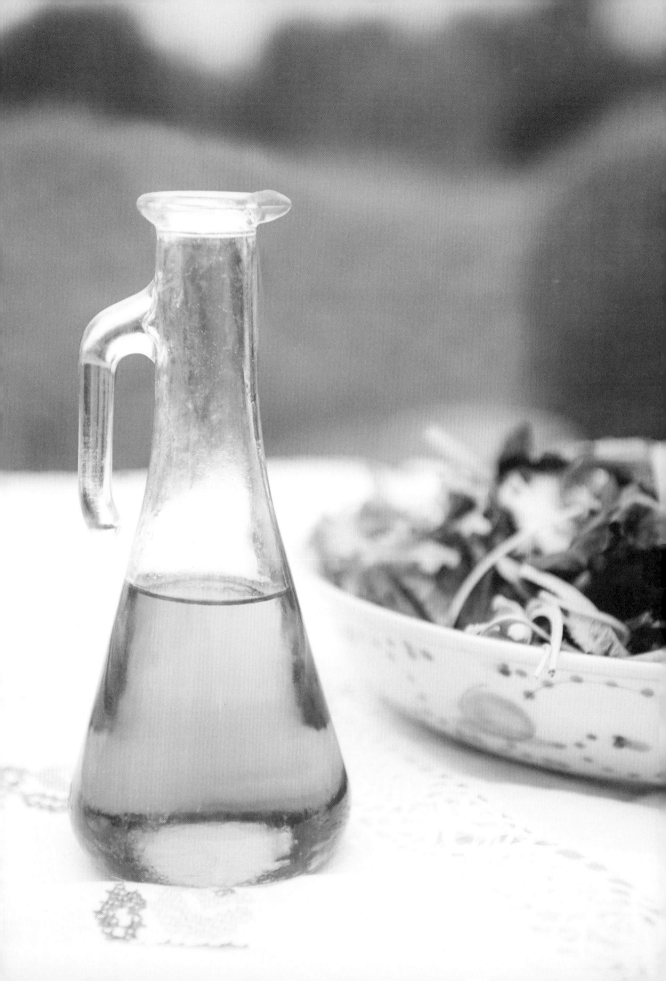

Lavender

Lavandula

Lavender reminds me of hot, dreamy summer holidays; hardly surprising, as it is a Mediterranean plant. It was bought to northern Europe by the Romans, they used lavender flowers in their communal baths, not just for the smell, but also to enjoy its antibacterial properties.

Along with chamomile, lavender is one of the best known plants for relaxation. This means that using the plant anywhere near bedtime is soothing and calming; a bunch under the pillow or near the bed is one way of inhaling its benefits. Lavender is also a mild antidepressant with its essential oil much loved by aromatherapists, so inhale this deeply to keep the blues at bay.

For the skin, lavender and rose used together in a bath are soothing after too much sun. Lavender also makes a good hair rinse for dandruff (see Nettle and lavender hair rinse). Owing to its antibacterial properties, lavender is good for treating minor cuts and sores; it is also antifungal, so it can help treat fungal infections such as athlete's foot or ringworm.

lavender footbath

This footbath is healing, antibacterial and antifungal, so it can help with athlete's foot or other fungal skin complaints on the feet. As an alternative to a footbath, put the cooled liquid into a spray bottle and spritz it onto affected areas; it will last for up to two days. (For more about the benefits of sage see the winter section.)

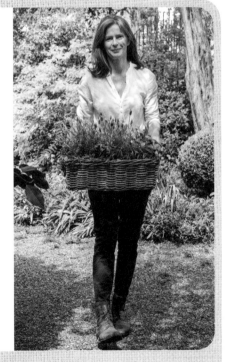

what you need

- 1 handful of lavender flowers
- 1 crushed garlic clove
- 3 torn sage leaves
- Water to fill the pan
- Small pan

1. Fill the small pan with water then add the lavender flowers, garlic and sage leaves.

2. Bring to a gentle simmer for 10 minutes, stirring.

3. Then take off the heat and drain out the plants, keeping the liquid.

4. Let the liquid cool, then add to a footbath.

5. Soak feet for 10 minutes.

recipe

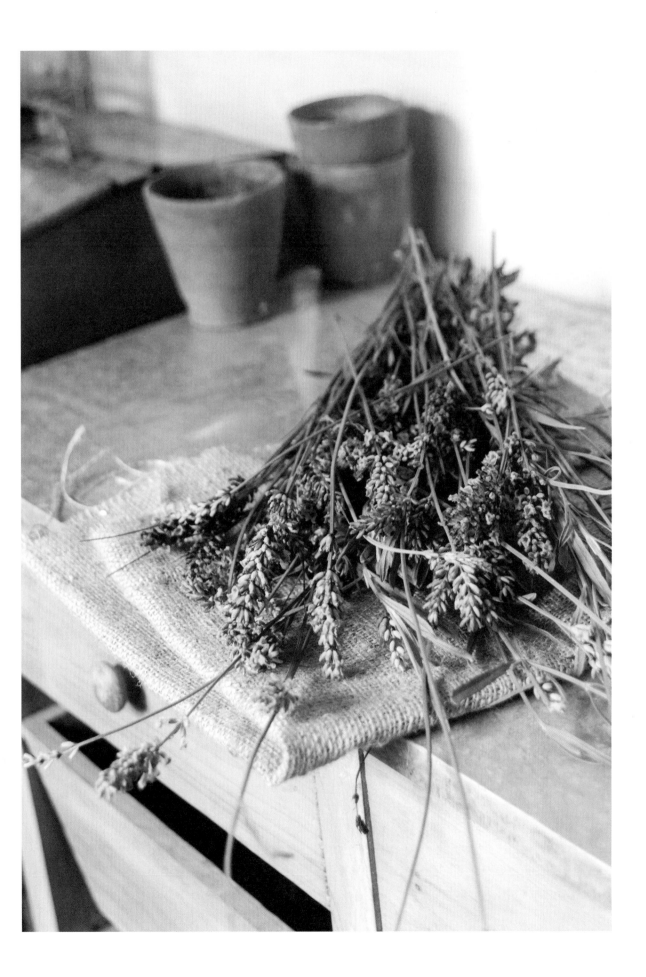

lavender bath bomb

This recipe is fun to make with children, as it is almost like building mini sandcastles. These bath bombs make bath time 'fizzzz' and the lavender not only smells heavenly, but along with the bicarbonate of soda (baking soda), works to soothe the skin.

what you need

- 300g (10½oz) bicarbonate of soda (baking soda)
- 100g (3½oz) citric acid
- 50ml (2fl oz) sunflower oil
- 2 dessert spoon (24ml) lavender petals
- 30 drops of lavender essential oil
- Greaseproof (wax) paper
- Bowl and metal spoon
- Small moulds such as ice cube trays, cookie cutters or cupcake shapes, even half a ping pong ball works!

1. Put all the dry ingredients in a bowl and mix them together with a metal spoon.

2. Pour the sunflower oil over the mixture and stir it in well; you need to achieve a consistency like wet sand, so if it is too dry add a splash more oil. Then add the drops of essential oil.

3. Now spoon the mixture out into your moulds. This process is rather like making mini sandcastles: pat the contents of the moulds down well with the back of a teaspoon – the firmer the better – then tip your bath bombs carefully out onto the greaseproof paper.

4. Leave them to dry on the greaseproof paper, which will absorb any of the excess oil. In a few hours they will be dry to the touch and ready to use, or leave them overnight for a really firm bath bomb.

5. Pop them in your bath and watch them 'fizzzzz'! Or if you want to keep them, put them in an airtight container to exclude any moisture and they will last for a month or two.

Sot SAYS... The bath bombs make great presents: to finish, put them in a little cellophane bag tied with a ribbon.

A word of caution: this recipe uses citric acid, which is like a form of manufactured lemon juice. Be very careful when using it, as it can irritate your skin and eyes; if you do get citric acid in your eyes, wash it out immediately. Also take care when handling the lavender essential oil, as it is strong and can irritate some people's skin.

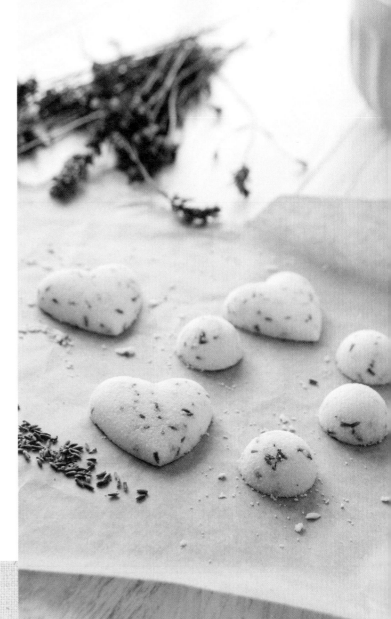

recipe

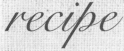

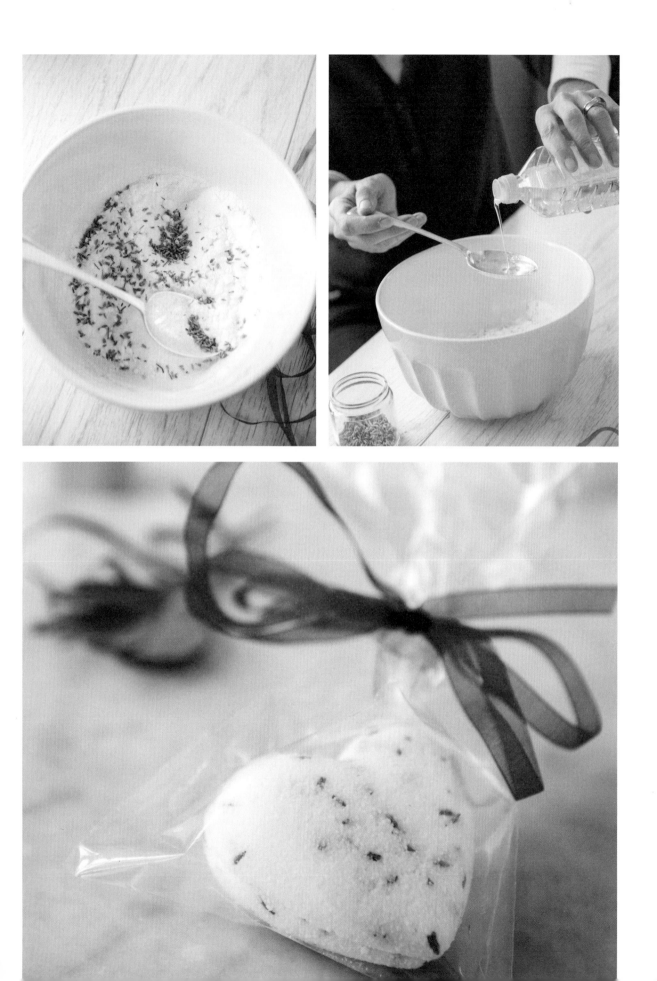

Lady's Mantle

Alchemilla vulgaris, alchemilla mollis

These plants are easily recognizable: I love their lime green flowers and large clumps of leaves, often seen with a small pool of water in the leaf centres as their saucer shape catches the summer rain. They are not 'wild' as such, but once established they keep on growing and spread very easily. These plants emerge in early summer, but if you cut them back they keep going right through the season, regularly pushing out new growth.

USES FOR LADY'S MANTLE

Lady's mantle (alchemilla) has been in use medicinally since medieval times, when folklore says it was given its common name after the Virgin Mary's mantle, or cloak, which its scalloped-shaped leaves are said to resemble. When dealing with wounds, alchemilla is known to have a particular affinity with stopping bleeding. Indeed, the great medieval herbalist Nicholas Culpeper wrote of alchemilla in 1653: 'It wonderfully dries up all humidity of sores and abates inflammations therein'.

The ability to dry and heal wounds is due to the plant's high tannin content, which makes the plant naturally antiseptic and able to inhibit bacterial growth. Tannins are also mildly astringent on the skin, so alchemilla makes a good toner, protecting the skin's elastin. Alchemilla leaves can be used in an infusion for a mouthwash to help bleeding after dental work; just let the infusion cool then rinse your mouth with it. The plant also has affinities with hormonal conditions and a tea made of alchemilla is thought to help with excessive menstrual bleeding.

A tincture of alchemilla leaves can be added to balms to soothe dry cracked hands and feet, or the leaves can be added to baths to calm the skin.

According to the English plantswoman Jekka McVicar, the species of alchemilla vulgaris (or xanthochlora) has more potent medicinal properties than alchemilla mollis, although it is perfectly acceptable to use either for your treatments.

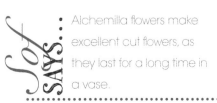

Sof SAYS… Alchemilla flowers make excellent cut flowers, as they last for a long time in a vase.

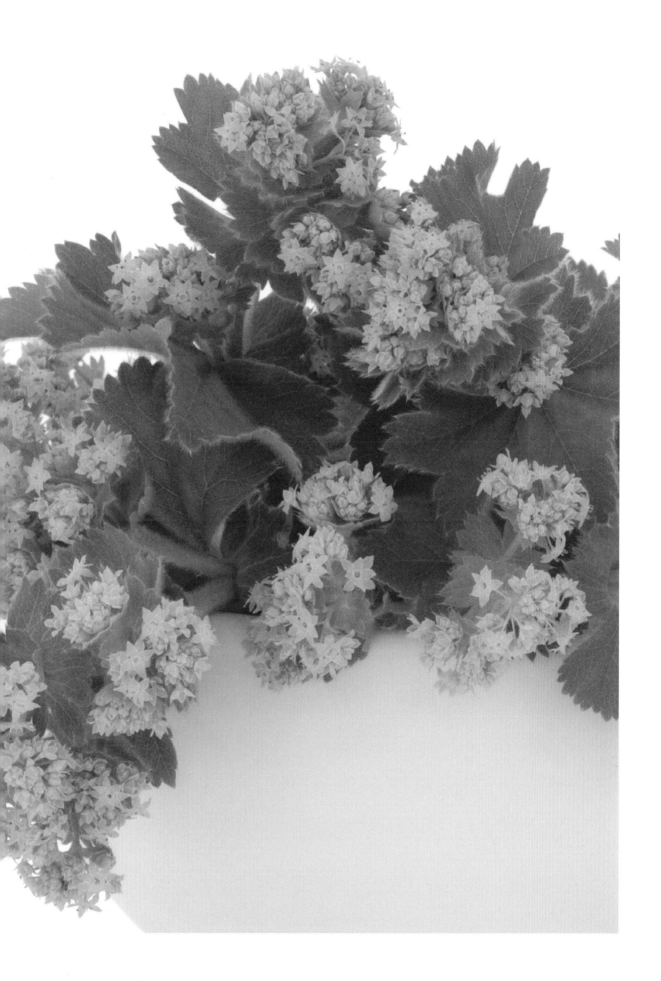

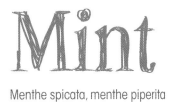
Mint

Menthe spicata, menthe piperita

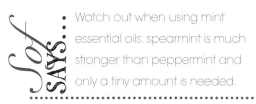

So says... Watch out when using mint essential oils: spearmint is much stronger than peppermint and only a tiny amount is needed.

Most of us are familiar with mint for use in the kitchen, with its fresh sweet taste and distinctive aroma. However, used outside the kitchen it is wonderful too. There are several different kinds of mint around that have similar qualities; applemint, spearmint and peppermint to name a few. Spearmint is stronger than peppermint, and it is peppermint that is more widely used.

When planting mint, watch out as it spreads via its roots and can soon take over a plot. It is best to grow it in a container sunk into the ground to stop it spreading or drying out, as it also likes moist conditions. If your plant does take over, late summer is the time to chop it back and use it fresh, or dry it for winter use; you can never have enough mint in the home.

Peppermint is classified as a carminative, which means it relieves intestinal wind, hence its use as a digestive aid. Just pop a few fresh or dried leaves in a mug and pour boiling water over them, perfect to drink after you have eaten a rich meal.

Due to its menthol content mint has a cooling effect, so it's good for easing hot, tired feet and itchy skin by putting a handful of leaves in a footbath (see Lavender footbath). To refresh your face in the summer, try making your own a facial mint spray: just pour some boiling water over a handful of leaves, let this infusion cool, then put it in a spray bottle to use when needed. As mint contains tannins and is antibacterial, your spray will also tone your skin, helping to restore elasticity, tighten pores and reduce any redness.

mint oil

This is a quick way to make an oil from plants.

what you need:

- 5 handfuls of mint leaves, stalk and all
- 500ml (18fl oz) sunflower oil
- Pan
- Seive

1. Put the mint and oil in th epan, making sure that the oil covers the mint, if not add more.

2. Heat this up slowly for 2 hours, on the lowest heat if you can – do not let it even simmer

3. Drain to remove the leaves and keep the oil that will last for six months; you can use it for cooking, too.

recipe

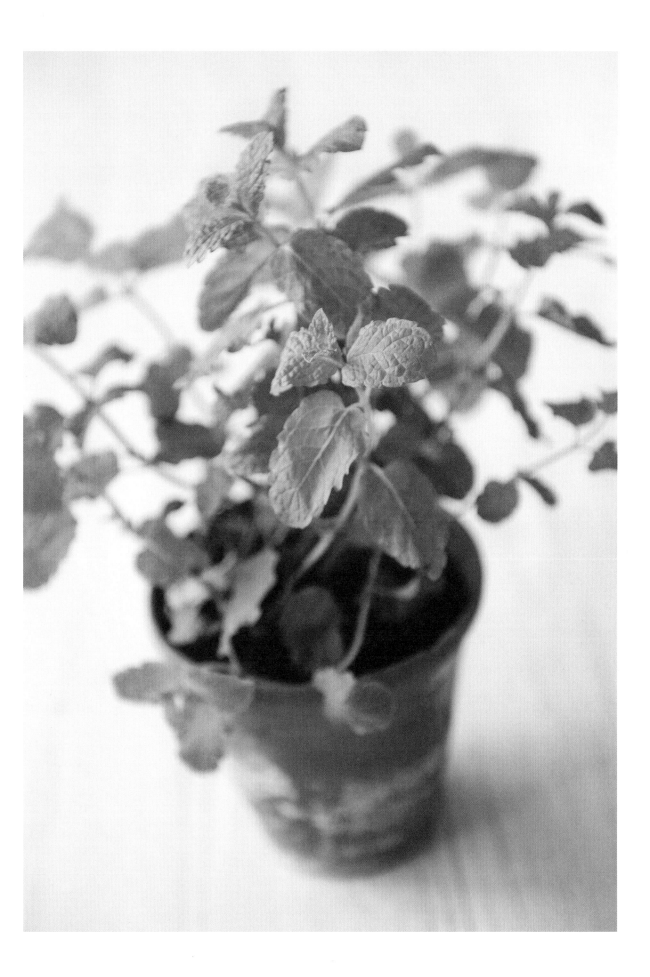

mint lip balm

This lip balm will make a wonderfully soothing balm to use over the summer months: the smell of mint on the lips is refreshing and the cocoa butter in the balm nourishes dry lips. If you don't want to make your own mint oil, use plain sunflower oil along with a few drops of mint essential oil or natural mint food flavouring instead.

what you need

- 25ml (1fl oz) homemade mint oil or sunflower oil
- 9g (¼oz) beeswax
- 12g (½oz) cocoa butter
- 4 drops of peppermint essential oil, or natural oil-based mint food flavouring (only needed if you have used plain sunflower oil)
- Small, clean pot with lid that will hold approximately 50ml (2fl oz)
- Small pan, with a lip if possible
- Kitchen paper (paper towels) for wiping up any excess balm mix

1. Put the mint oil or sunflower oil, beeswax and cocoa butter in a small pan and gently heat until all the ingredients have melted. It is very important to do this gently and slowly; do not simmer at any point.

2. Once the mixture has melted, take it off the heat and add the essential oil or food flavouring if you have used plain sunflower oil.

3. Now pour the mixture into your pot, put the lid on and leave to cool for 30 minutes. An important note: if you spill any of the mixture, use kitchen paper for wiping it up, and wipe your pan with kitchen paper before washing. Do not pour down the sink, as beeswax can block the pipes as it hardens.

4. Once cooled, label and use. That's it – it really is super easy!

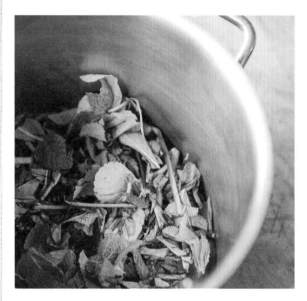

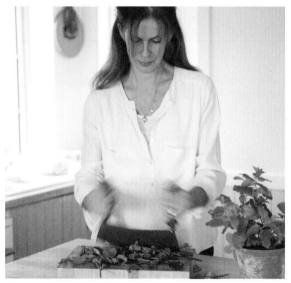

LIP BALM VARIATIONS:
- If you want a shinier, glossier lip balm, replace the mint or sunflower oil with avocado or castor oil.
- If you want a more healing lip balm, use home-made marigold oil instead of mint oil.
- If you want to make a nourishing hand balm, just follow this recipe and add homemade rose petal oil instead of the mint – it will smell divine.
- If you want a lip balm for cold sores, replace the mint oil with lemon balm oil (*melissa officinalis*), which is antiviral.

recipe

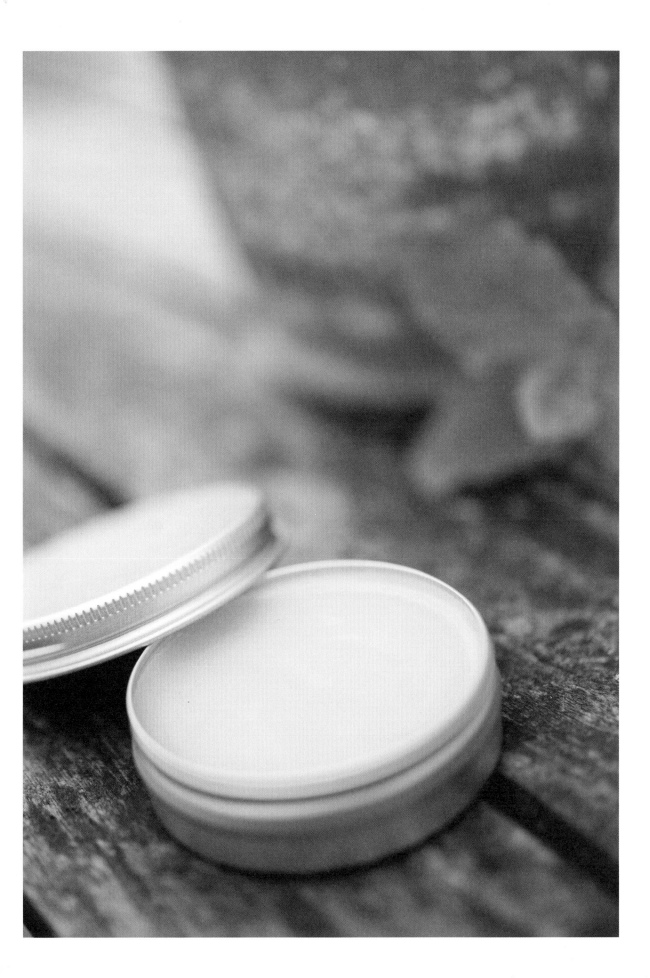

Harvesting Plants

Apart from picking plants for their beauty and smell, summer is the time of year to be harvesting them for use throughout the coming winter months. I once visited a herb drying farm where they had custom-built sheds for drying the plants, with wooden slatted shelves up each wall and heated pipes underneath – the smell in the lavender shed was incredible! But don't worry, harvesting and drying can be done at home on a much smaller scale. Throughout this book there are many ideas and recipes that call for fresh or dried plants, and by harvesting and drying your own you will always have a ready supply to hand.

CHOOSING YOUR PLANTS

First you need to choose and pick the plants you want to dry. For **flowers**, good options are lavender, rose petals, marigold or yarrow; for **leaves**, choose mint, nettles or artemisia. Try to pick specimens of these plants in good condition, not ones that have 'gone over'. You then need to dry the plants, without them becoming a damp pile of rotting vegetable matter, or reducing them to dried out crisp crumbs. Warmth and circulating air are crucial, so it is best not to attempt to dry too many plants at once.

DRYING YOUR PLANTS

There are various methods you can use to dry the plants:

*   You can lay them on newspaper on a tray and leave them somewhere warm and dry. A sunny window sill is perfect.
*   Or you can place them on racks on a very low oven heat; you can even keep the oven door open, so they don't turn crisp.
*   Or you can hang the plants upside down to dry, allowing air to circulate freely around them.
*   If you have space in your airing cupboard, this is a good place to dry them.

Once dry, put them in a clean airtight jar so you can use them all year; on average most will last for a year, but some will last longer, like mint.

Jo says... Dry hydrangeas by hanging them upside down to keep as much colour in the flowers as possible; these will look great in the home all winter. You can only dry these flowers towards the end of the summer; any earlier and they will just wilt.

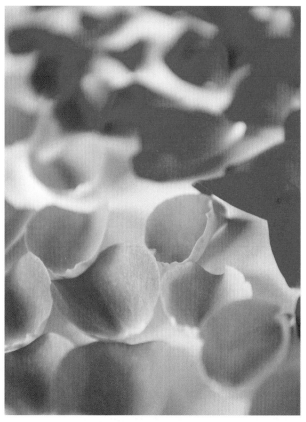

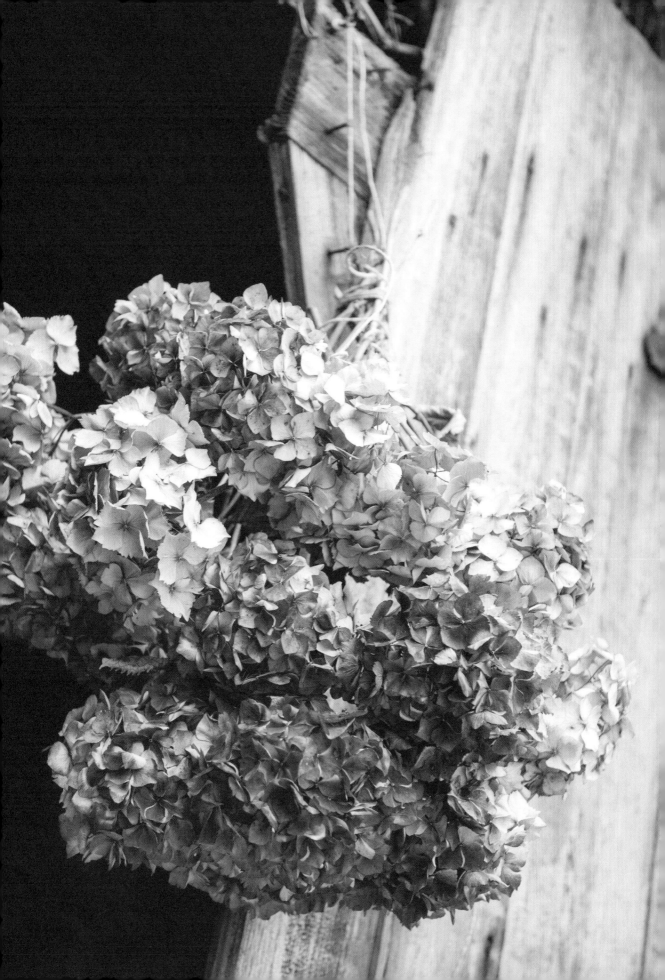

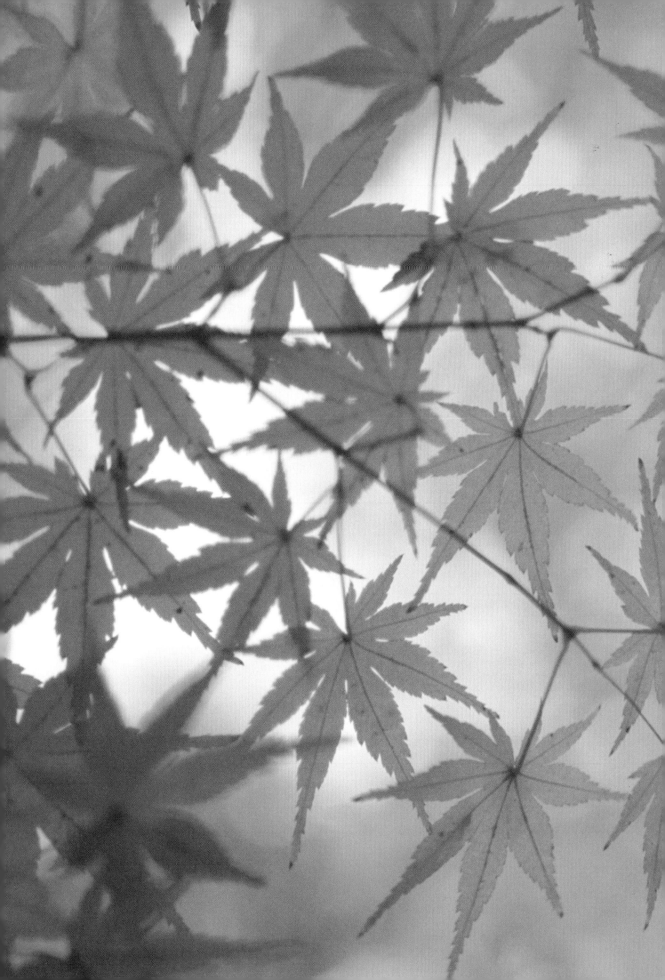

autumn

As the leaves start to turn and a crisp chill creeps into the air, Mother Nature's health store is filled to the brim with vitamin-rich berries. From the bright red of rose hips to the glossy black of elderberries, now is the time to get gathering and make your own pre-winter tonic. A word of caution: if you do go berry picking, be sure you know what you are collecting, as there are poisonous berries ready to fool us. It is also the season for bonfires and Halloween, so at the same time Nature offers us a variety of ready remedies for burns and shocks.

Contents:

lemon verbena: calming yet refreshing tea
rose hip: syrup packed with vitamins
beetroot: juice to help the heart
hedgerow spirit: a good glug to keep you going
conkers: veins and pains
hawthorn berries: hearty tea
burns: for seasonal bonfires

bumps and bruises: So you can keep moving
elderberries: the perfect winter tonic
monkshood: a poisonous cold beauty
blackberries: a classic autumn jam
wormwood: keep away those nibbling moths
rowan berries: just juicy jelly
witch hazel: an all-round remedy

Lemon Verbena

Aloysia citrodora, aloysia triphylla

This plant originally derives from South America and loves the sun, thriving in a warm, well-drained soil. At first glance, it may not seem an obvious choice to include here, but it is pretty robust and has managed to grow in my damp, wet English garden. I think it is definitely worth the effort of growing your own lemon verbena, as its leaves make my favourite tea of all, sometimes known as vervain tea. You just need to make sure you plant lemon verbena (*aloysia citrodora* or *aloysia triphylla*), and not *vervain officinalis*, which does not make a relaxing tea to drink.

When young, lemon verbena is a small plant, which means it can be grown in a pot on a sunny windowsill. The fresh leaves have a light lemony scent, not unlike old-fashioned lemon sherbet sweets. You can harvest them throughout the summer, but early autumn is your last chance to stock up for winter. Once cut, the leaves dry quickly if left in the sun for a few hours, a process that slightly softens the smell. Store the dried leaves in an airtight container where they will keep for up to three years for you to use when needed.

USES FOR LEMON VERBENA

The leaves are slightly antifungal and antibacterial, yet I think their best use is for making a relaxing lemon verbena tea. This is soothing and calming to drink in the evening; it is also a good digestive tea that relaxes the gut. The main component in these leaves is an essential oil known as citral, which is used in the perfume industry to create a fresh lemony scent. Lemon verbena leaves contain about 30 per cent citral, whereas the leaves of Australian lemon myrtle contain over 90 per cent. It is this citral that makes lemon verbena so good to cook with: add it to jellies and puddings to bring a subtle lemon tang to your dishes.

Just use a bit of caution when using this plant, as some people are allergic to citral oil.

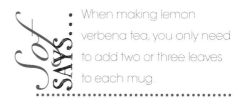

Sot SAYS... When making lemon verbena tea, you only need to add two or three leaves to each mug.

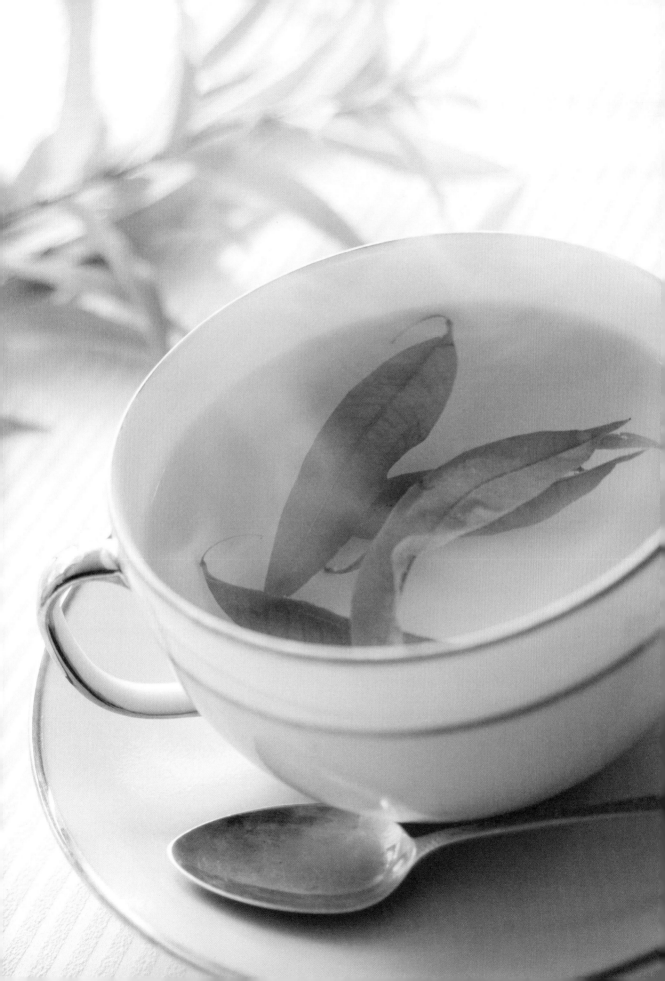

Rose Hip

Rosa canina.

So **SAYS...** If making rose hip tea, watch out for the fine hairs around the pips; careful straining to remove them is required.

Rose hips – or haws – are fruits of the common wild dog rose, and are not only a vital seasonal food for birds, but are also of great benefit to us. Country lore says that rose hips are better when they have been softened by the first frost, but don't wait too long to pick them or they will become shrivelled husks. It has been known for a long time that rose hips contain high amounts of vitamin C to provide a much needed winter boost, and traditional recipes for rose hip jams, jellies and syrups are widespread. With fewer wild areas, finding wild rose hips is harder these days, so you may need to plant your own or buy dried ones.

Their high levels of vitamin C make rose hips ideal for helping to fight off colds and winter bugs; try making a refreshing cold-fighting tea using the dried fruits. They also have anti-inflammatory properties, which may be beneficial for joint pain; indeed two Scandinavian studies into chronic joint conditions revealed reduced pain and increased motility following a course of rose hip supplements. Rose hip oil is a dry oil (see Oils) and is good for repairing damaged skin, for calming sensitive skin, and for fighting skin infections such as blackheads.

what you need

- 1 small cereal bowl of fresh rose hips to make 500ml (18fl oz) of syrup
- 1 litre (1¾ pints) water to cover the rose hips
- 100g (3½oz) caster (superfine) sugar
- Small pan
- Sieve lined with muslin
- Clean bottle or jar
- Optional: 1tsp (5ml) citric acid, if required as a preservative

rose hip syrup

Making rose hip syrup is a wonderful autumn activity, using the ruby red hips that you have collected on an autumnal walk. As the seasons turn your syrup will come into its own to boost vitamin C levels and to help ward off colds.

1. Shake out your collected rose hips, put them in the pan and cover them with water.

2. Bring this to the boil then reduce the heat and leave simmering for half an hour, periodically mashing the fruit with a fork or potato masher to release all its goodness, and topping up the water if needed.

3. Drain the mixture into a clean pan through a sieve lined with muslin, squeezing out all the juice you can. Keep the liquid and discard the rose hips.

4. Add the caster sugar to this liquid then gently heat again to dissolve all of the sugar.

5. If you have citric acid, add a spoonful now so the syrup will last longer. This is not essential, as the rose hips have a high amount of vitamin C that does a similar job of preservation.

6. Pour the syrup into a small bottle or jar and take one or two teaspoons a day throughout the coming months.

recipe

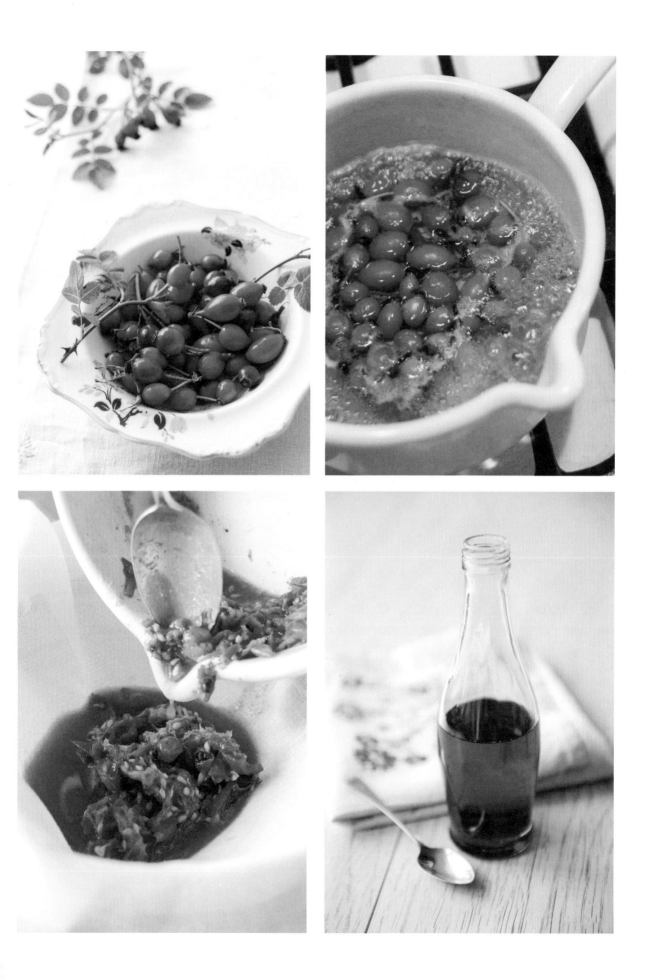

Beetroot

Beta vulgaris

In autumn there is often a glut of beetroot, making this the ideal time to stock up on this versatile root vegetable. You could even offer to take some off the hands of any gardening neighbours; you never know, if you ask you may get lucky! It has taken me a while to come to love its taste, and I know that it is either a 'love it or hate it' vegetable. If you love it you are really in luck, because it is very good for you.

Beetroot is full of antioxidants and nutrients such as magnesium and betalain; the latter is important in many metabolic processes in the body, especially in the heart and liver. Beetroot also has a high nitrate content, which means it will lower blood pressure. Indeed, recent research has revealed that drinking less than 300ml (½ pint) of beetroot juice a day will help lower blood pressure levels.

The pigment in beetroot is known as betanin: it is strong and it stains, which is why it is used as a food dye. In addition, the body is not easily able to break down this pigment, so it is excreted in urine, turning it the colour pink.

EATING AND DRINKING BEETROOT

Making a simple beetroot juice is a great way to obtain your beet goodness. Roughly chop and blend the beetroot in a juicer, then add a chunk of ginger for a spicy kick, as well as a squeeze of lemon to stop the juice from tasting too sweet.

Another way to consume beetroot is to make a delicious beetroot, onion and apple chutney; probably not as full of goodness as the juice due to the sugar content, but at least it lasts all year. Making any chutney is very easy: simply cut up the ingredients, then boil them with sugar and vinegar, and in this case a little ginger and garlic.

You can try adding finely grated beetroot to salads for a healthy lunch, or make a traditional borsch (beetroot soup). This is one of the easiest soups to make: peel and chop beetroots, carrots, onion, garlic and celery; simmer in a good stock; then blend and serve. This really is my kind of cooking, as just one pan is used!

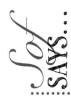

Sof SAYS... Whole roasted beetroot is an easy way to eat beetroot; just add a little olive oil and a pinch of salt.

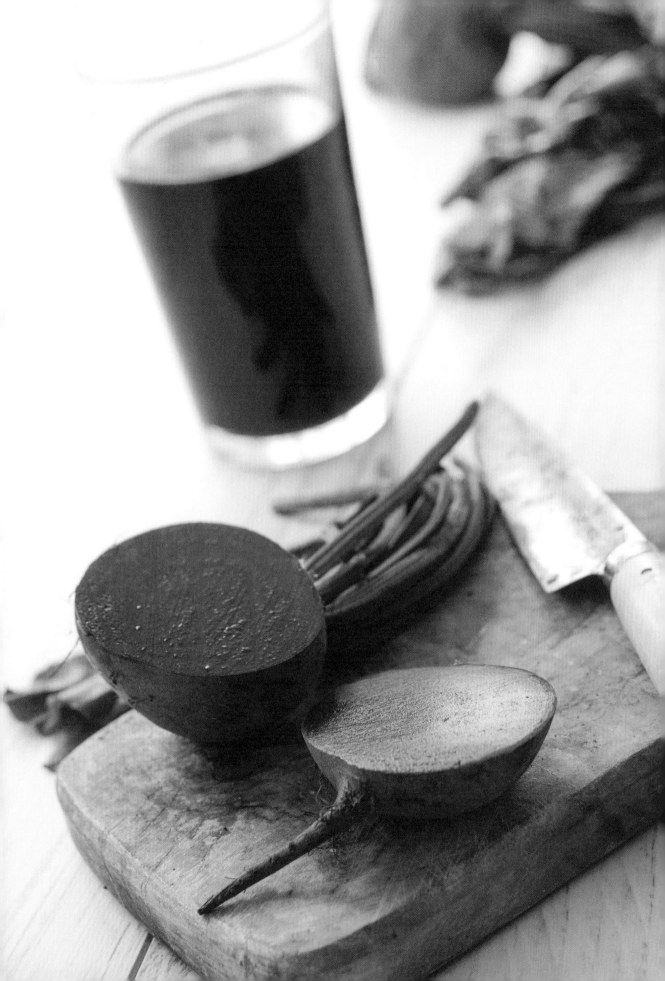

Hedgerow Spirit

I could write about the health giving properties of the fruit you will add to this alcoholic beverage – but really that is insignificant compared to the delicious taste and the fun you'll have making a "hedgerow spirit". If you don't fancy making it for yourself, prepare some now for great Christmas presents, as the fruit needs time to soak. I promise, you will be very popular during the festive season!

For this recipe you can use whatever fruit you like; I have even tasted rhubarb vodka. In the wild, sloes and damsons often alternate yearly, so one year you will find trees laden with fruit and the next year you'll find none. Here are some tried-and-tested fruits to make your spirit with:

- **Damsons** are my favourite, with a rich, sweet flavour. They are small purple-blue plums with a stone inside, but larger than sloes.
- **Sloes** come from the blackthorn bush (*prunus spinosa*), which is common in hedgerows. They are small, dark fruits and less sweet than damsons, so need more sugar.

- **Blackberries** can be used to create a dark, sweet drink (see Blackberries).
- **Blackcurrants** (*ribes nigrum*) are full of many health benefits and are packed with vitamin C. They make a tangy but sweet tipple; they are the berries used to make crème de cassis and the sweet Ribena drink.

Whichever alcohol you use, don't waste money on anything expensive as the fruit will add so much flavour. Gin is either a 'love it or hate it' choice with its juniper berries and other botanicals already giving it a distinctive flavour, whereas vodka is more or less just pure alcohol. You could use rum, although I find it too sweet.

hedgerow spirit

This is an easy recipe and the quantity you make depends on the amount of fruit you harvest.

what you need

- 1 bottle of alcohol, 700ml (70cl)
- 50g (2oz) fruit of your choice
- 25g (1oz) caster (superfine) sugar, or 37g (1½oz) if using sloes
- Large wide-necked sterilized jar, or several smaller ones if you can't find a large one
- Bottle for the finished product

1. The skin on the fruit is best broken, so either prick it with a fork or put it in the freezer so the skins burst a little. As a note: the freezer option is best if using small berries like sloes and blackcurrants; neither option is needed if using blackberries, as they are so soft.

2. Once this is done, place the fruit in large sterilized jars that have wide enough necks to drain the fruit from at the end of the process.

3. Pour your chosen alcohol over the fruit then add caster sugar.

4. Shake vigorously immediately, then store in a dark place for two or three months; during this time shake again whenever you remember to do so.

5. After two or three months, strain off the alcohol into sterilized bottles, and let them sit for a time. Your spirit will improve with age, lasting for a long time.

Sof SAYS… Instead of throwing away any fruit, use it with apples to make a wintery fruit crumble. Or add it to melted dark chocolate, pour into moulds and leave to set to make your own delicious chocolate bar. This makes a great present, but remember that it contains alcohol.

recipe

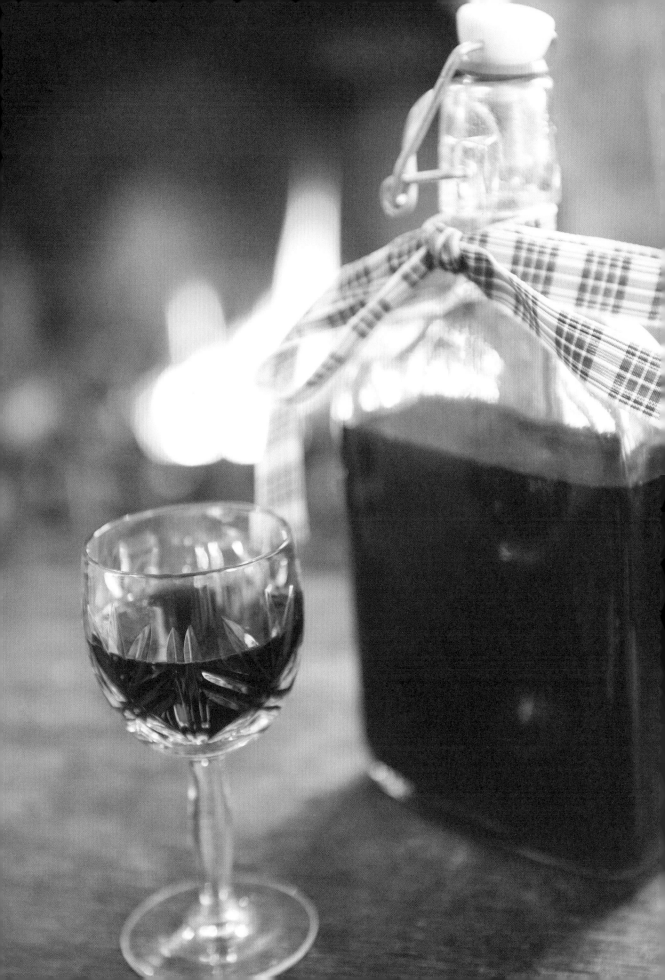

Conkers

Aesculus hippocastanum

Autumn is the time to gather up shiny conkers from the ground; after an early morning walk in the park I come home with bulging pockets full of them. Conkers are the nuts of the horse chestnut tree, a large striking tree with candelabra-style flowers that grows easily in temperate climates as far north as Norway in Europe and Alberta in Canada. Conkers should not be confused with the delicious edible chestnuts that come from the sweet chestnut tree (*castanea sativa*).

Conkers contain aescin that works on the elasticity of blood vessels, helping to restore strength to them; this has a positive effect on the flow of blood. Indeed, studies have shown that aescin can help treat varicose veins, thread veins and piles. Conkers are also rich in the natural anti-inflammatory quercetin, which is good for swollen painful joints, and they are used in the homeopathic remedy aesculus to treat painful haemorrhoids.

MAKING CONKER TINCTURE

Make a conker tincture by grinding the nuts then seeping them in alcohol for two weeks (see Tinctures). Cutting the conkers can be hard work, so use a coffee grinder or a sharp bladed blender to help you do this. This tincture can then be applied externally by adding it to a plain base cream, or by adding a few drops to a balm or ointment base (see Balms and Ointments). A word of caution: this homemade tincture should not be used internally.

Remember always do skin sensitivity test first.

 Sof SAYS... Here is a tip from the College of Naturopathic Medicine in the UK. Carry two or three horse chestnuts removed from their conker shells around in your pocket to help relieve arthritis pain. When the nuts become dried up and hard, replace them with fresh ones.

conker skin toning ointment

If you have made your own conker tincture, this recipe is ideal for using it in an oil-based ointment that you can rub into your skin where you need it most. If you've not made your own tincture, you can purchase a ready-made one.

what you need

- 15g (½oz) beeswax
- 20ml (½fl oz) sunflower oil
- 70ml (2½fl oz) calendula oil
- 10ml (¼fl oz) conker tincture
- 5 drops of lavender essential oil
- Small pan
- Small, clean pot, approximately 110ml size

1. Melt the beeswax and sunflower oil in a small pan very slowly on a very low heat.

2. Remove from the heat then add the calendula oil, which is excellent for skincare.

3. Now add the conker tincture, stirring or whisking well to make sure the alcohol is mixed; then add the lavender essential oil for a nice smell.

4. Pour the ointment into a small, clean pot to rub into your skin nightly.

recipe

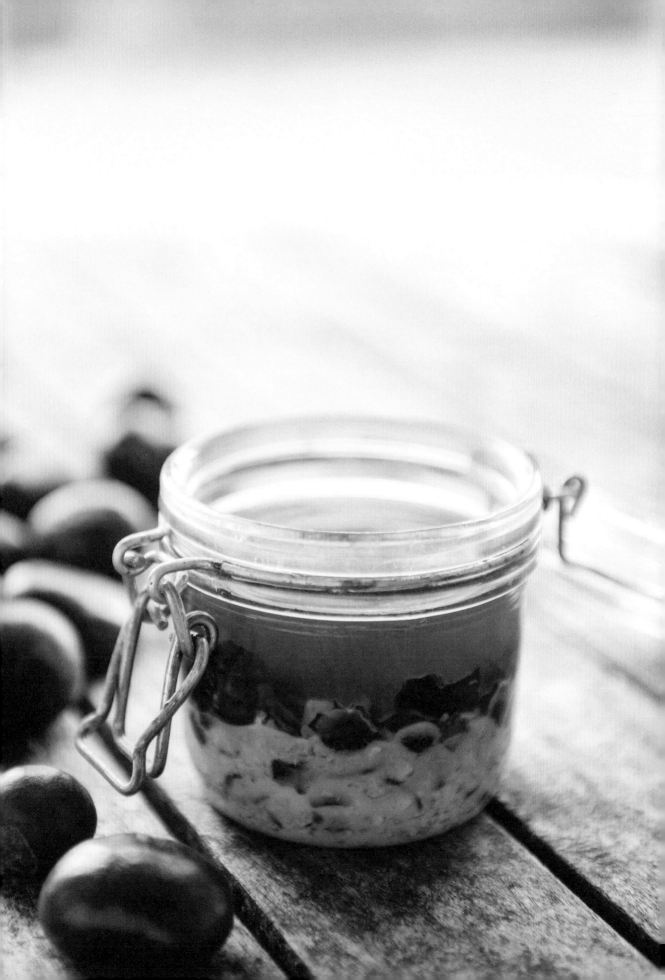

Hawthorn Berries

Crataegus laevigata, crataegus monogyna

Hawthorn is one of the most common hedgerow plants found in northern temperate climes, providing an effective thorny barrier for farm animals. Its old name 'May flower' tells us when the flowers bloom, and in autumn the berries are ripe for picking. If you can't find any growing near you, purchase dried hawthorn berries from health food shops. Medicinally the berries – or haws – are good for many things, but if you only remember one, remember its use for the heart and all aspects of the circulatory system.

The berries are now well known for their properties in helping to regulate blood flow and the early stages of some heart problems. They can also ease some conditions that are caused by poor blood flow in the arteries such as Raynaud's disease, which is where circulation to the extremities is impaired, often leaving the finger tips temporarily blue.

To use hawthorn to treat these ailments, try making a tea with either dry or fresh berries; leave it to steep for at least 10 minutes before drinking so you glean all the goodness from the berries. Alternatively, try making a syrup (see Elderberries); as the berries are full of pectin, the syrup will be nice and thick.

chewy berry leather

For something a bit different, why not try making a 'leather'? This can be done with most berries; other good choices to use for this recipe are rose hips and cranberries, although only use a little sugar with the latter if you want them to help with cystitis. Eat a square measuring approximately 2cm (¾in) across a day.

what you need

- Berries of your choice
- Water to cover the berries
- Caster (superfine) sugar to taste
- Juice of 1 lemon
- Pan to fit the berries
- Baking tray (sheet)

Sof SAYS... Hawthorn is also good for easing menopausal mood swings.

1. Put your berries and sugar in the pan with water just covering them.

2. Simmer them for 15 minutes then boil for a further five minutes.

3. Take off the heat and coarsely blend the berry mixture.

4. Add the lemon juice then spread the mixture in a thin layer on a baking tray.

5. Cook in the oven on a low heat: 110°C (225°F/Gas Mark ¼) for two hours.

6. After cooking, peel from the baking tray then break up and store in jars.

As with any home remedy, never self-treat if you have a serious condition or are on medication; this is especially the case with hawthorn as it contains heart-affecting compounds. Also never take it in large amounts as it can cause dizziness and low blood pressure.

recipe

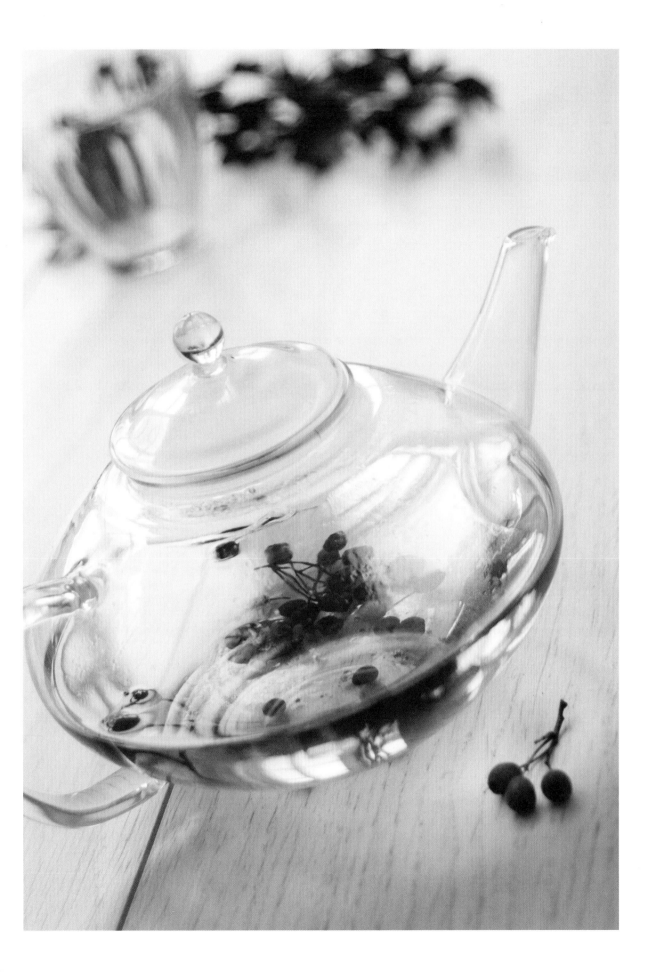

Burns

This is the season of bonfires, so it is a good idea to have a few remedies to hand during these darkening autumn days to treat minor burns. Please remember that serious burns require urgent medical help and need to be immersed or held under cool running water until that help arrives to reduce pain and swelling. Don't remove any clothing if it has become stuck to the skin; and don't apply any creams or gels.

If the burn is minor or superficial then it can be soothed with several plant-based creams or gels:

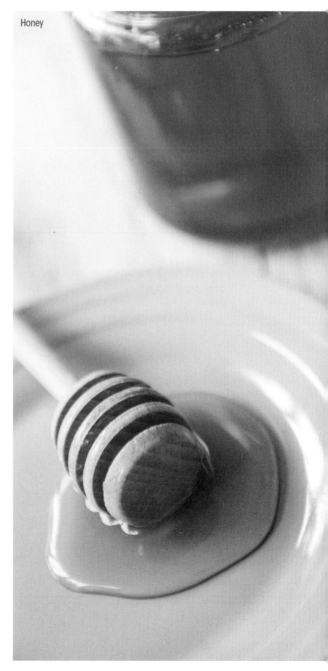

Honey

- **Aloe vera** is a favourite of mine and a tropical plant, but even in northern climates you can grow one as a houseplant. For minor burns just break off a leaf, cut it in half, and apply the clear gel that oozes from the centre directly onto the skin.

- **Witch hazel** is a well known astringent; packed with tannins, it soothes and tightens the skin (see Witch hazel).

- **Cantharis** is an excellent homeopathic remedy made from the Spanish fly that can relieve pain from burns, especially blistering ones. Cantharsis can be taken orally or applied as a ready-made cream; in the latter it is often combined with urtica – the common stinging nettle – which has a soothing effect.

- **Calendula** is pot marigold and is good for skin regeneration after a burn (see Pot marigold).

- **Honey** can be used, particularly manuka honey or medi-honey, which have more antibacterial properties than normal honey. Dab it on a burn very carefully.

- **Vinegar** can generally be found around the home and is useful in an emergency. It can soothe small minor burns if the skin is not broken, and is especially good for sunburn.

Bumps and Bruises

Some people are just clumsier than others, and I am one of them. I often find unexplained bruises on my legs, then remember I'd just walked into the edge of a table or door. Here are some ideas to help with minor bumps and bruises, or general muscle aches and pains.

Arnica has to be the flower of choice for minor bumps and bruises is a small yellow alpine belonging to the daisy family. Its old English name of 'fallherb' provides us with a clue as to its uses: for years herbalists have crushed the leaves to soothe bumps and bruises.

Arnica can be applied externally as a cream or ointment to help with bruising, swelling and tissue damage after falls, or aching, pulled muscles and sprains caused by excessive exercise. You can make your own infusion (with water) or tincture (with alcohol) from the leaves to use externally, but do not use on broken skin.

Arnica can *only* be taken internally in its homeopathic form, as the plant is very toxic. As a homeopathic remedy, it is highly diluted so none of the toxins remain. Take arnica as a homeopathic pill as soon as possible after a fall, before all the muscles seize up and the body goes into shock recovery – it can help the body process the bump. At times like this, I like to think of the body as a huge tuning fork: knock one bit out of shape and this reverberates throughout, yet the arnica somehow helps the body to re-organize itself.

Other remedies to consider for bumps and bruises:

* **Ruta** and **Rhus tox** are both plant-based homeopathic remedies that are good for injury and stiffness in joints and muscles.

* **Comfrey** used externally is good for bruises (see Comfrey).

* **Witch hazel** can be used externally on bumps when the skin is broken, but arnica and comfrey can not (see Witch hazel).

* Always get professional advice for serious bumps and bruises, or if the pain continues.

So says... Once muscles have seized up after a fall, a cold compress is crucial to reduce the swelling; for chronic muscular pain, heat pads are better.

EPSOM SALTS (MAGNESIUM SULPHATE)

A cup or two of Epsom salts can be added to a bath to soothe muscular aches and joint pains; use in this way after physical exercise to prevent muscles from stiffening up. Used in a bath like this, these salts are also known for drawing toxins out of the body and reducing swelling.

Internally, you can take Epsom salts to keep the bowels moving; as the expression goes, it went through me like 'a dose of salts'. Only a tiny amount is needed: just put half a level teaspoon in a glass of warm water, stir well and drink. It can act quite fast.

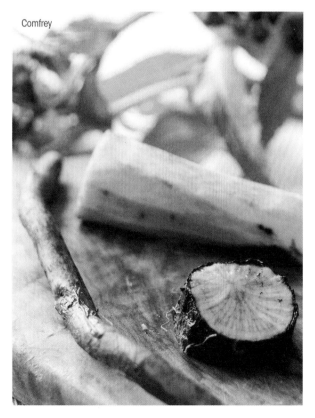

Comfrey

Elderberries

Sambucus nigra

Elderberries are from the elder tree, which we already came across in spring with its magnificent elderflowers (see Elderflower). Choosing the time to pick elderberries is a fine art: unlike rose hips and hawthorns that can benefit from an early frost, you can't leave delicate elderberries too late. So from early September onwards keep your eyes peeled; you want to pick the large saucer-shaped heads when they start to droop downwards heavy with ripe berries, not leaving them to become so ripe that the birds eat them all or they start to go over. Do note: while the birds eat these berries, it is not advisable for humans to eat them raw as they are mildly toxic and will cause stomach upset.

USES FOR ELDERBERRIES

Once you've picked your elderberries you can make jam, jelly or syrup with them. Anything really, as long as they are cooked. Making a syrup is a great way to get the goodness from the berries as they are packed full of vitamin C, as well as iron, calcium and potassium, all of which are good in a winter tonic.

You can buy elderberry syrup ready-made in chemists, often under its Latin name sambucus, but as even a small bottle can be expensive, it is a good idea to try and make your own. Sambucus is also the name for a homeopathic remedy used to treat suffocating night-time coughs and sweaty fevers accompanied by chills.

When using yarrow, be aware that most of the active ingredients are to be found in the flowers. These contain salicylic acid, which has pain relief properties and is the main ingredient of aspirin. Leaves are also used, but they are not as strong as the flowers.

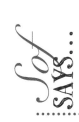

Sot SAYS...

The elder tree is one of my favourites – not only is it very robust, but you can harvest it twice a year, in spring and autumn.

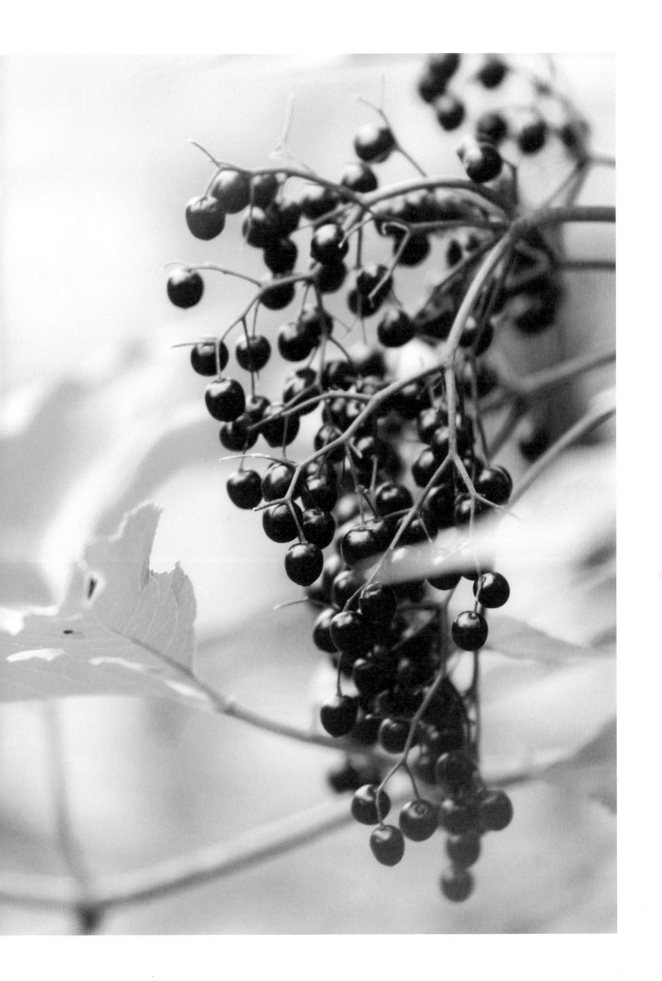

elderberry syrup

This syrup is perfect to drink throughout the winter months to boost your immune system and help keep colds at bay. You can take two teaspoons neat on a daily basis, or dilute the syrup to drink as you would a cordial; it is even delicious to pour over yoghurt and pancakes. Simply adjust the recipe quantities to the amount of berries you pick. The important measurement is not how many berries you use, but how much liquid you make from them after you have boiled them, as this will determine how much sugar and preservative to add.

what you need

To make approximately 3 litres (5¼ pints) of syrup:
- Approximately 7 litres (12¼ pints) fresh elderberries picked from their stems
- Approximately 2.5 litres (4½ pints) water (see Step 2)
- 600g (1lb 5oz) caster (superfine) or granulated sugar, depending on how much liquid you make (see Step 8)
- Either 60 cloves or 90ml (6 tbsp) citric acid for preservation, depending on how much liquid you make (see Steps 8 or 10)
- Bowl
- Pan
- Sieve lined with muslin
- Sterilized bottles or jars

1. Pick over the berries first, discarding any old or mouldy ones and cutting off the larger woody stems. Stripping them from the smaller branches is easy with a fork; don't worry too much if some small stems remain, as draining through muslin later will catch any debris.

2. Put all your picked-over berries in a pan then add cold water so it reaches just under halfway up the berries; any more and your syrup will become too watery.

3. Bring this to the boil, crushing and stirring the fruit from time to time.

4. Once it has started to boil, turn the heat down to simmer for 20 minutes, again stirring and crushing the berries from time to time. Then take off the heat and leave to cool.

5. Once cool, strain through a sieve lined with muslin into a large bowl. If you don't have any muslin a fine sieve will do an adequate job, but you will most likely find a few bits left in your liquid.

6. Leave the elderberry liquid to drip through the sieve and muslin; the process can be helped by putting a plate on top of the berries as an extra weight, or just push through with the back of a spoon.

7. If you don't want to waste any juice from the berries, squeeze out the muslin with your hands – you will be surprised how much more juice comes out. But be warned: the juice will stain your hands in the short term and is wonderfully messy!

8. Measure this liquid to determine how much sugar to add: 200g (7oz) of sugar per one litre (1¾ pints) of liquid. If you are adding cloves as a preservative, you need 20 cloves per one litre (1¾ pints) of liquid. Remember that these will affect the taste, too.

9. Return the liquid to a clean pan, add the sugar and gently heat up the elderberry liquid, stirring so the sugar dissolves. Bring to a gentle simmer for five minutes.

10. Take off the heat, and if you are using citric acid instead of cloves, add two heaped tablespoons of citric acid per one litre (1¾ pints) of liquid. Stir in well so it is all dissolved.

11. Now pour your liquid into bottles or jars using a funnel if necessary, and sieving out the cloves if you have used them.

12. Then label and use. Your syrup will last for three months and is best kept cool in the fridge, or you can freeze it.

recipe

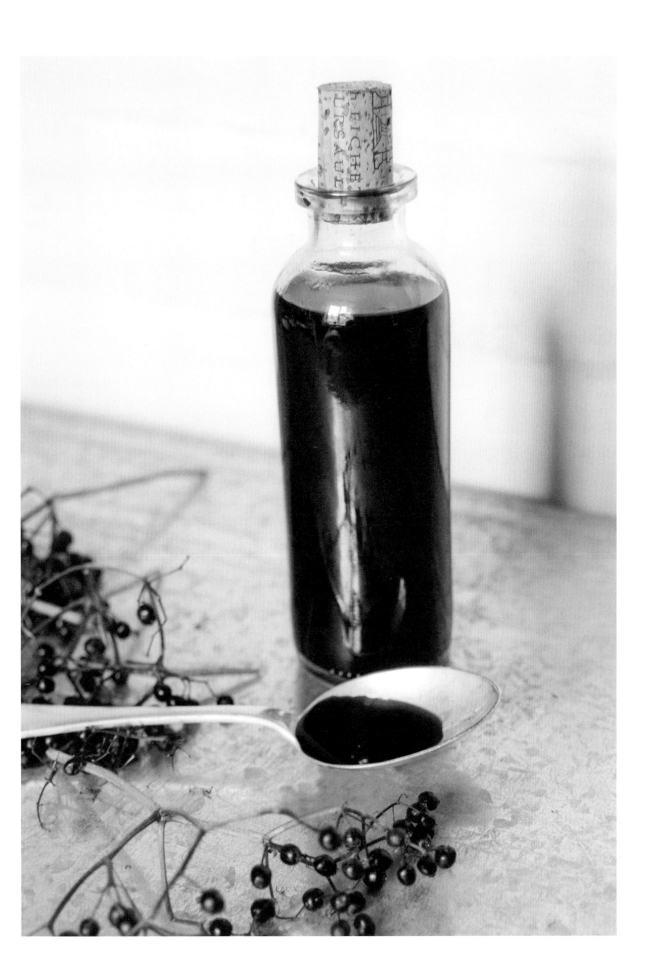

Monkshood

Aconite

This poisonous flower blooms well into the autumn season, so it adds a fine touch of colour to autumn gardens. Furthermore it also useful for treating shock, just in case those ghouls and ghosts on Halloween prove a little too scary! This plant is in the 'poisonous' section of my medicinal garden. I planted a couple of bulbs and for a long time they did nothing, but patience paid off and in October their tall, striking forms rose above the other plants, and their elegant dark blue heads provided some much needed colour when all else faded.

Monkshood (aconite) is one of homeopathy's best cold remedies. If you take homeopathic aconite at the very first sign of a cold, it will often nip it in the bud, especially if the cold came on suddenly. Homeopathic Aconite is a good remedy for shock, or for the distress caused by a frightening event. It is often helpful in sudden labour where there is a fear of being unable to cope; it *certainly* helped with my very fast two hour labour, in which I was like a 'rabbit caught in headlights'!

HOMEOPATHY AND POISONOUS PLANTS

Homeopathy has a long history of using poisons in its medicines, by taking miniscule amounts and diluting them further and further. This is always done in a laboratory and is **never** to be done at home. Other poisonous plants that are made into homeopathic remedies are:

- Belladonna or deadly nightshade, which is good for fevers.
- Arnica (see Bumps and bruises), which is good for bruising.
- Digitalis or foxglove, which is good for heart weakness.
- Rhus tox (see Bumps and bruises) or poison ivy, which is good for joint and muscle aches, and used to ease the itch of chicken pox.

 An important warning: monkshood – or aconite – can ONLY be used as an expertly made homeopathic remedy, highly diluted and reduced to non-toxic levels in a laboratory. Every part of the plant is highly poisonous, and for that reason it has been dubbed 'the queen mother of poisons'. Indeed, another name for it is 'wolf's bane', as hunters used it on the tips of their arrows to kill wolves. So please never make your own home remedy from this beautiful plant.

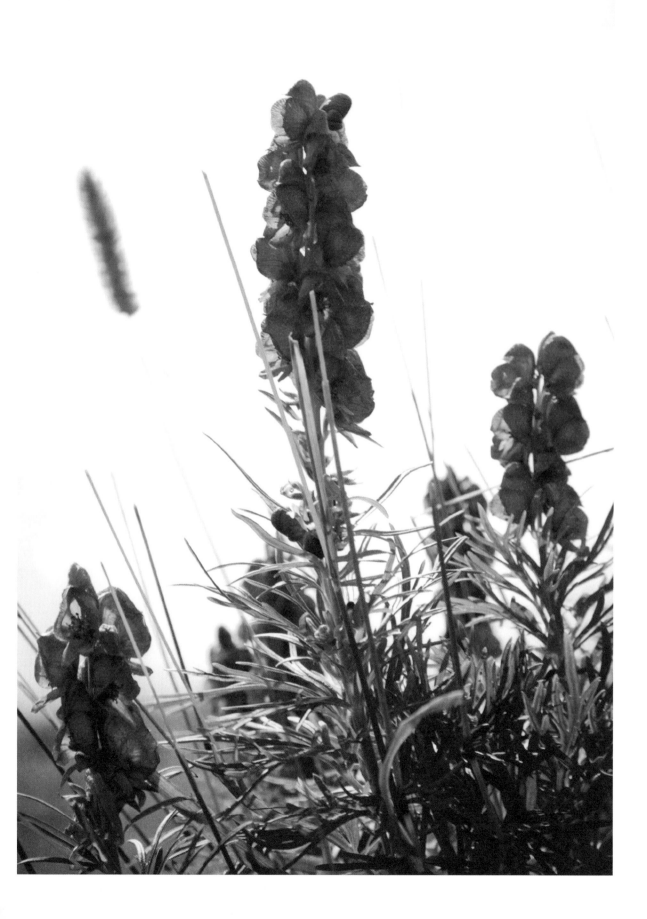

Blackberries

Rubus fruticosus

These familiar berries are found in hedgerows from late summer through to early autumn and are the one fruit that many people will have foraged for. They make a welcome addition to any home remedy store – if you can gather enough without eating them all first.

Blackberries are full of antioxidants, so they help fight off colds and generally boost your immune system. Some antioxidants occur naturally in our bodies, but their effectiveness decreases with age, so replenishing stocks through our diet is beneficial.

Blackberries are also full of manganese, which is an essential trace mineral and necessary in all living organisms; for us it is great for bones and general cell function. Too much manganese is toxic, but don't worry: this relates more to excessive supplementation or inhalation of manganese in the mining and metalwork industries, rather than overdoing it while blackberry picking!

blackberry and apple jam

There is nothing as nice as making and storing blackberry and apple jam to provide a taste of autumn throughout the winter months. This recipe makes approximately eight jars of jam; I like the half-sugar-to-fruit ratio (described here), as you can really taste the fruit rather than the sugar, although you may need to keep opened jars in the fridge as they won't last so long.

what you need

- 1.5kg (3lb 5oz) blackberries
- 500g (1lb 2oz) chopped apples (weighed after being peeled and cored)
- 1kg (2lb 4oz) preserving sugar
- 200ml (7fl oz) water, to reach halfway up the fruit in the pan
- Large 5 litre (10 pint) pan
- Jam thermometer (if available) or 4 chilled saucers
- Sterilized jam jars
- Waxed discs, lids and labels

1. Put all the ingredients into the pan, squashing the fruit a little with the back of a spoon.

2. Slowly heat, making sure all the sugar is dissolved, then increase the heat to boil and continue a rapid, rolling boil for seven to nine minutes; you are aiming to reach a setting point for the jam of 104°C (220°F).

3. If you have no thermometer, do the saucer test after eight minutes of boiling. Using a cold saucer (from the fridge), drop a little of your jam onto it, let it cool for a minute, then push it with the back of a spoon or your finger to see if it will wrinkle. If the surface of the jam does wrinkle it is set; if not, continue boiling and try again in a few minutes.

4. Pour or ladle the jam into the jars (a large metal funnel can help with this) and wipe up.

5. Put the wax discs onto the jars (wax side down) while the liquid is still hot, to ensure a good seal and to help the jam last longer. Then put on the lids.

6. Wait until the jars are cool then label. Unopened jars will last for six months to a year, if you don't eat them before that!

recipe

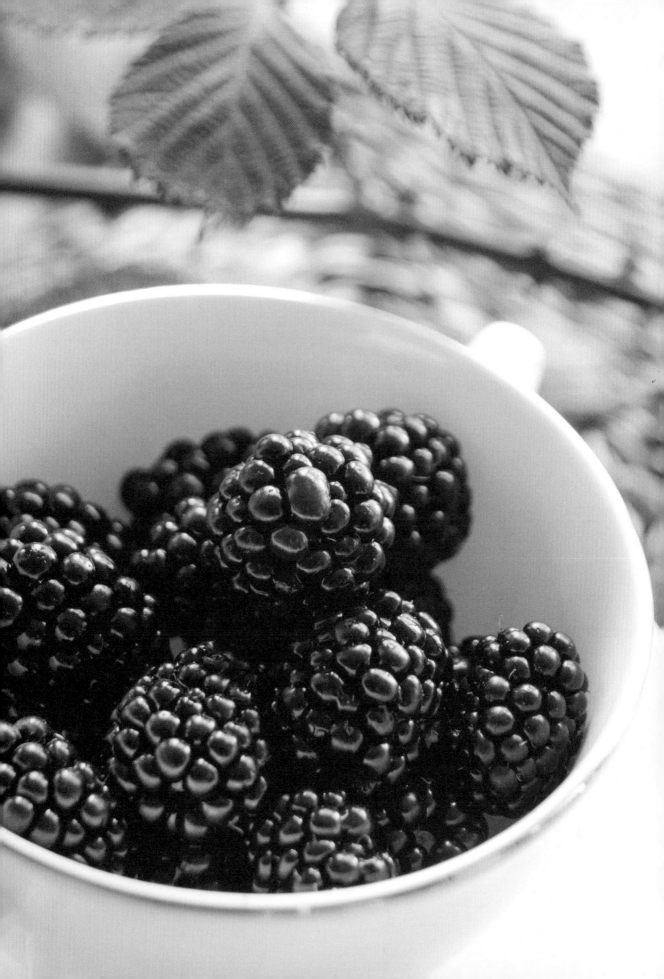

Wormwood

Artemisia absinthium

Wormwood – or artemisia – with its lovely silver foliage is beautiful in any border; it prefers well-drained soils, but is nevertheless pretty robust. If you plant it in Spring, it will quickly establish itself so you won't have to wait long to harvest. As its name suggests, wormwood is a herbal remedy for internal worms, but I don't recommend that you use this unless under professional care as it can be toxic. However, it is far more accessible for use as a moth repellent, and I have recently planted it specifically for this use. Some related plants are: southernwood (*artemisia abrotanum*) with its green delicately scented leaves, which is also a good moth repellent and bunches can be hung in the kitchen to deter annoying flies; and mugwort (*artemisia vulgaris*), which is an ancient magical healing herb.

MAKING INSECT DETERRENTS

Pesky cloth-eating moths are often the scourge of warm modern homes, as they can now breed throughout the year to happily feed on your woollen jumpers and silk shirts. To make a moth deterrent to combat this damage, cut several large bunches of wormwood leaves and flowers in early Autumn and hang them upside down to dry. Once fully dried, hang them in your wardrobe or place them in your cupboards; the smell of the wormwood will deter the moths. If you are feeling creative with a sewing machine, you could even make up some small cloth bags in which to put the crumbled dried leaves – perfect additions to drawers. The plants will work for about two months or whenever the smell has sufficiently deteriorated.

Some other plants that can be used to repel insects are as follows:

- Rosemary and sage can be dried and added to wormwood sachets to help repel moths.

- If you have an ant infestation, rub pennyroyal on the surfaces where the ants are.

- For dog fleas, try rubbing tansey (*tancetum vulgare*) and rosemary into the dog's coat and bedding.

- To deter flies, hang up bunches of tansey and wormwood.

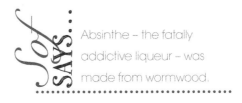

Sol SAYS… Absinthe – the fatally addictive liqueur – was made from wormwood.

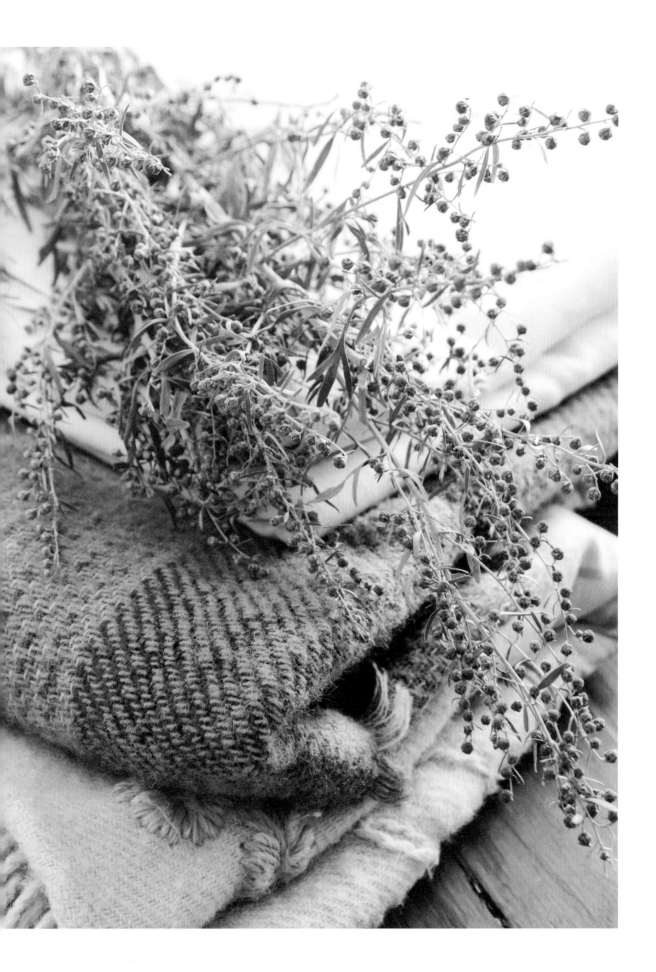

Rowan Berries

Sorbus

The rowan tree, or mountain ash, is a hardy deciduous tree that thrives in northern climes. There is much folklore and mysticism surrounding rowans, and according to my mother – who is very practical and not mystical at all – every garden should have a rowan tree for good luck. I have included these berries, not so much for their health giving properties, but more for their free abundance, as they make a delicious jelly that gives a good tang to any roast meats.

rowan jelly

This jelly is delicious with any meat or cheese, but particularly with game and venison, perhaps owing to the wildernesses where wild rowans grow. The quantities you use in the recipe depends on the number of berries you pick; after boiling and draining them, just measure the resulting liquid to determine how much sugar to add. No pectin is needed to help the jelly set, as the berries are rich in this substance. After making, leave the jelly for a couple of weeks before you eat it; the taste of rowan is too bitter at first, only later do the subtle flavours develop.

what you need

- Rowan berries, picked over with any large woody stems removed
- Water to reach halfway up the berries in the pan
- Granulated sugar
- Large heavy-bottomed pan
- Sieve lined with muslin
- Measuring jug
- Jam thermometer (if available) or 4 chilled saucers
- Sterilized jam jars
- Waxed discs, lids and labels

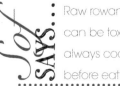

Sof SAYS... Raw rowan berries can be toxic so always cook this fruit before eating

1. Put all your berries in the pan, then add cold water to reach halfway up the berries. Bring to the boil then let the mixture simmer away. As it does so, stir and crush the berries to the side of the pan with a wooden spoon to make a soft mush; if this looks too dry, just add more water.

2. After about 20 minutes, or when the berries are all soft and cooked, drain them through a sieve lined with muslin, keeping the liquid. If you want very clear jelly, leave the liquid to slowly drip through the sieve; however if you are not bothered about the clarity, push it through with the back of a metal spoon to extract every last drop .

3. Measure your liquid and pour it back into a clean pan, adding sugar. The rule of thumb is that for every 1 litre (1¾ pints) of liquid, you need to add 800g (1lb 12oz) of sugar. You can add more, but bear in mind that rowan jelly should have a naturally bitter, almost acrid tang, very different from sweet redcurrant jelly.

4. Heat up slowly so the sugar dissolves, then cook this on a rolling boil for seven to ten minutes until it reaches a setting point of 104°C (220°F), all the while skimming off the scum. I keep this and eat it the same day so not to waste it; it still tastes delicious.

5. If you don't have a jam thermometer, do the saucer test instead: after boiling for eight minutes take a saucer from the fridge, drop some liquid onto it and let it cool for a minute. Then push it with the back of a spoon or your finger to see if it will wrinkle. If the surface wrinkles, it is set; if not, continue boiling and repeat the test in a few minutes.

6. Put the wax discs onto the jars (wax side down) while the liquid is still hot, to help the jam last longer.

7. Then put on the lids and label. The jelly will last for years unopened, probably due to it high levels of sorbic acid.

recipe

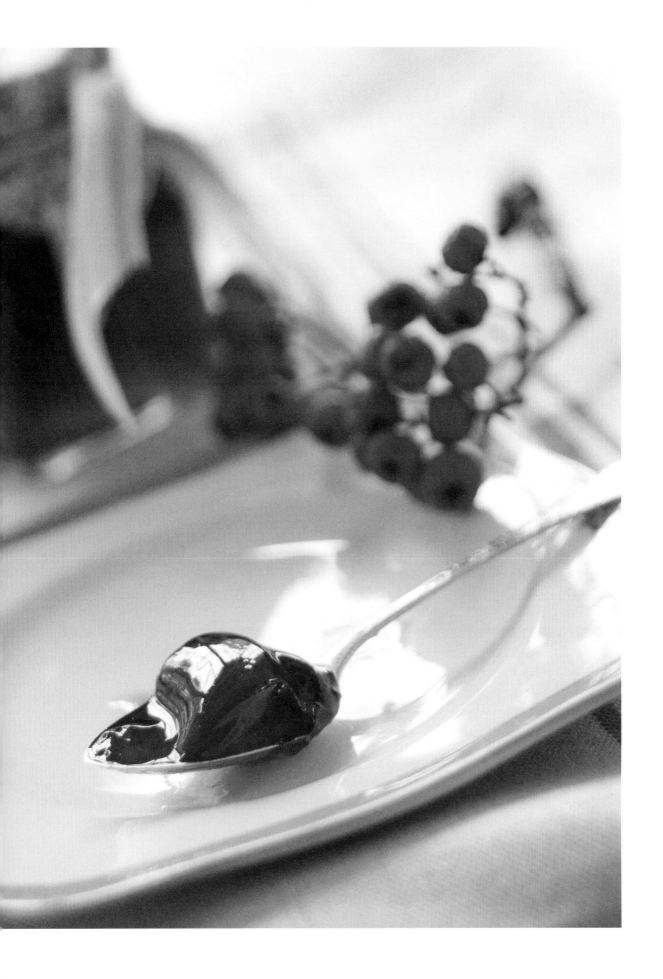

Witch Hazel

Hamamelis virginiana

The unassuming shrub or small tree is a wonderful source of goodness. You will probably only notice it in autumn when its small, bright yellow flowers come out, distinguishing it from a multitude of other small leafed shrubs. Other shrubs from the hamamelis family flower on bare branches in the wintry depths of January, such as Chinese witch hazel (*hamamelis mollis*). The Native Americans have long used witch hazel for its anti-inflammatory properties, passing their knowledge onto European settlers when they arrived.

Witch hazel has astringent qualities due to the tannins it contains and is great for many skin complaints; drying up troublesome spots and reducing inflammation, as well as being good antiviral treatment for cold sores. The same astringent action can also help to contract the swelling of varicose veins, piles and minor capillary problems. Witch hazel can help to ease the discomfort of minor burns and insect bites; it can also soothe the pain of bumps and sprains. In addition, it is also good to use in a hair rinse (see Nettles).

Only external use of this plant is recommended. The parts used for remedies are the fresh leaves and small twigs, and these can be used to make either a tincture infused in alcohol (see Tinctures), or as a decoction boiled in water (see Decoctions).

witch hazel spot gel

This recipe makes a strong gel to put on individual spots only, as it is very drying. Always carry out a skin sensitivity test before using.

what you need

- 40ml (1½fl oz) water
- 40ml (1½fl oz) homemade witch hazel decoction (2 tsp (10ml) of tincture)
- 1 tsp xanthum gum
- 5 drops of tea tree oil
- 5 drops of lavender essential oil
- 12 drops of Preservative 12, used in the vegan food industry in Denmark
- Small, clean pot, approximately 80ml size

1. First add the witch hazel decoction to the water.

2. Sprinkle on the xanthum gum, whisking it in well so there are no lumps.

3. Add five drops of tea tree oil for its antibacterial properties then five drops of lavender essential oil for its lovely smell and antibacterial properties.

4. Then add 12 drops of Preservative 12 if you want the gel to last, if you don't use this, the gel will last for a week.

5. Pour the gel into a small pot and dab it on a spot when you need to.

recipe

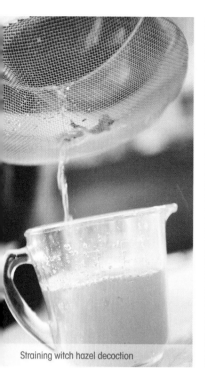
Straining witch hazel decoction

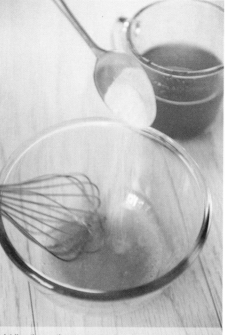
Adding the xanthum gum powder

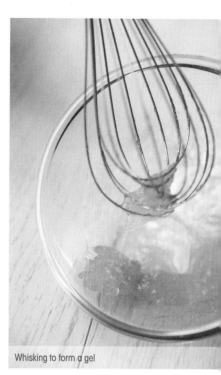
Whisking to form a gel

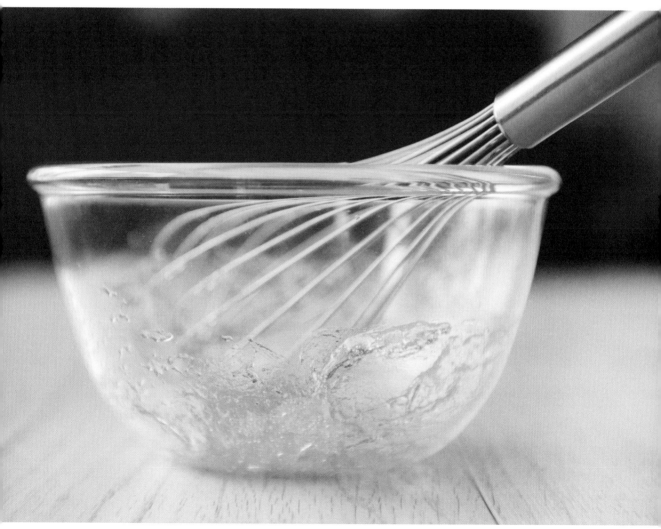

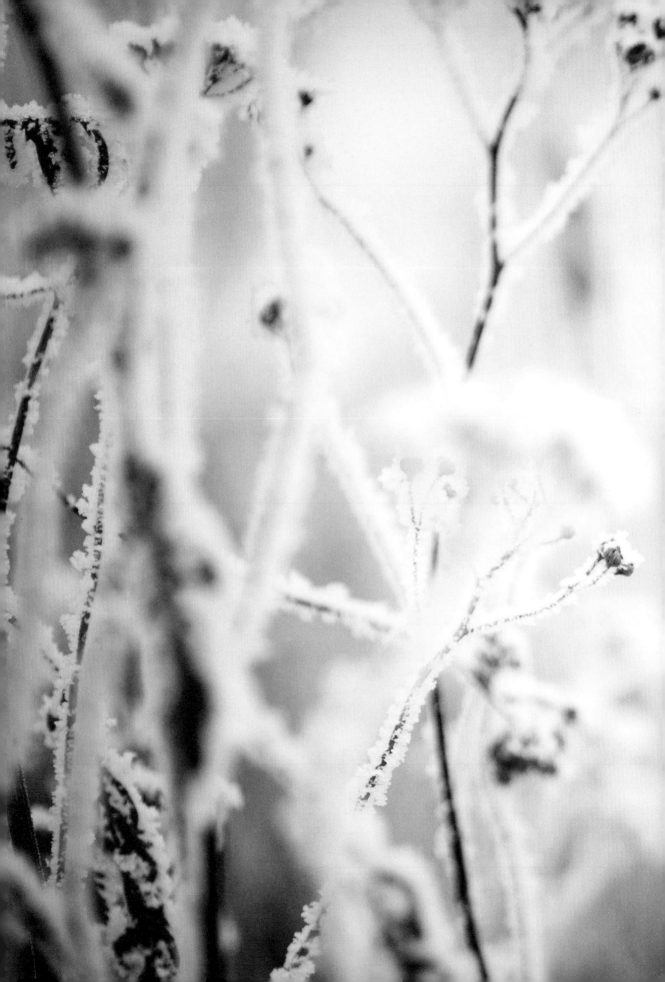

winter

As the nights grow longer and the days draw in, now is the time to hunker down and make the most of what you have gathered over the year. Don't worry if you didn't collect much; there are still many evergreen herbs available to use, such as rosemary and sage. This is also the time of year when the kitchen spice rack comes into its own: cinnamon, ginger and cloves all make great cold busting remedies for this busy season.

With the cold winter days this is a fantastic time of year for indoor activities and making presents is a fun way to keep out of the cold. Try making ginger chocolates, relaxing bath salts or invigorating body scrubs. Whatever gifts you choose to make, adding a personal label and a pretty ribbon makes all the difference, so let your creativity run wild.

Contents:

rosemary: remember me?
garlic: keeping your lungs free
sage: skin toner saver
overindulgence: soothing stomach ideas
cinnamon: curb those sugar cravings
ginger: chocolates with a zing

cloves: pretty pomanders
skincare: plants that are good for skin
body scrub: revive your skin
colds: how to treat them
bath time: restore and relax

Rosemary

Rosmarin officinalis

This well-known evergreen herb is perfect to use at this time of year as not only is it antibacterial to ward off winter colds, rosemary also has a myriad of other uses, from aiding memory to muscle relaxation, so it is well worth picking now, and being evergreen it is still going strong.

USES

- **Coughs and colds:** It's antibacterial, antifungal and antiseptic so will help with a huge range of coughs, colds and respiratory infections. Use in a steam inhale. (see picture)

- **Relaxation:** For joint and muscle pain use rosemary essential oil diluted in sunflower oil and rub on to the affected parts. Or make your own 'macerated oil' (see Mint). To relax the digestive system drink a tea of fresh rosemary, this encourages enzymes for food absorption so helping cramps and wind.

- **Memory tonic:** As the old song goes 'Remember me to one who lives there, parsley, sage, rosemary and thyme'. Rosemary has been called the herb of remembrance as it is thought to boost memory. Again a tea is good for this.

- **Skin:** As a topical ointment it can boost circulation and elasticity of the skin and help with dull oily skin and blackheads. Rosemary has a large amount of antioxidants, which reduce the effect of oxidation in the body. Oxidation produces 'free radicals' which are thought to contribute to ageing. Many natural health products have a rosemary extract in to naturally prolong its shelf life. It is also good as an external ointment for hard to heal wounds, dab an infusion of the leaves on the skin.

- **Hair:** You'll often see it in shampoos and conditioners, as it is good for dandruff and maintaining a healthy scalp. You can make your own rosemary hair rinse, just pour boiling water over crushed fresh or dried rosemary, leave to seep for half an hour, drain and use after shampooing, massaging into the scalp. Said to be good for stimulating new hair growth. (See Nettles)

Sof SAYS... Prolonged use of rosemary is not recommended, and the herb should never be used during pregnancy due to a risk of miscarriage.

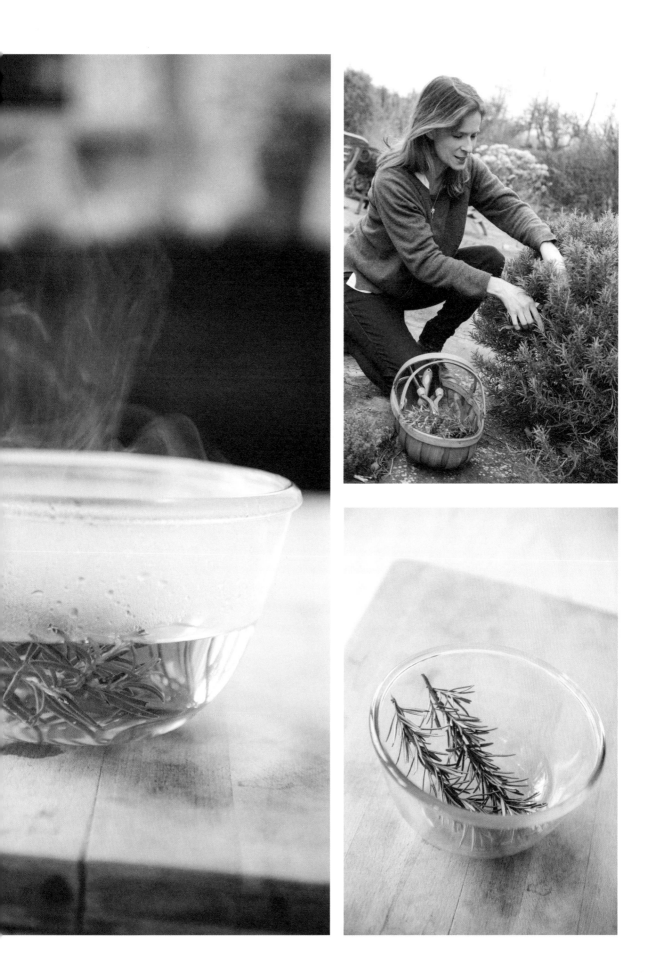

Garlic

Allium sativum

The garlic bulb really comes into its own at winter time with its powerful antiviral, antibacterial and antifungal properties. The active component here is allicin, which is released when the cloves are crushed or chopped; the bulb is also full of vitamins and minerals.

Because of these properties, garlic makes a great cold-fighting remedy, not just keeping them away, but also for reducing the duration of colds when you do catch them. Garlic is also beneficial for heart health as it may lower cholesterol levels and reduce blood pressure. However a word of caution: garlic also has certain blood thinning properties, so it is not advisable to use if you are already taking blood thinning medication.

Odourless garlic capsules can be bought to make the most of these benefits, but it is much more fun to increase the use of this versatile bulb in your cooking. Use it raw crushed in salad dressings, or cooked in tasty stir-fries, adding it near the end of the cooking process so that it maintains its goodness.

garlic and onion expectorant

At this time of year, when the cold weather makes us hunch up and winter bugs can settle on your chest, it is a good idea to keep everything moving. So here is a great garlic and onion-based expectorant to help promote the elimination of phlegm. It was given to me by herbal practitioner, Jill Davies from Herbs Hands Healing. The recipe combines the health giving properties of garlic with onion, another potent antibacterial bulb, which is also thought to initiate actions in the body that break up mucous congestion.

what you need

- 2 organic peeled white onions
- 1 organic peeled head of garlic
- 1 tbsp freshly grated or dried horseradish or 2 tbsps from a jar of horseradish relish
- 3 of the hottest organic chillies you can bear
- Approximately 20 organic black peppercorns
- 1 litre (1¾ pints) organic cider vinegar

1. Put all the ingredients in a blender and chop until you have produced a fine consistency.

2. Pour this into several large jars and leave to steep for at least two days; the longer you leave it, the stronger it becomes.

3. If it is too strong, you can add juice or honey to the mixture, although I think it is good to make the most of its savoury and hot nature.

4. Take a teaspoon of this when you need to, as it is good for colds, influenza and deeply rooted coughs; you can even add it to salad dressings.

 Sot SAYS...

Try eating a bunch of parsley after eating raw garlic, as this takes away some of the smell!

recipe

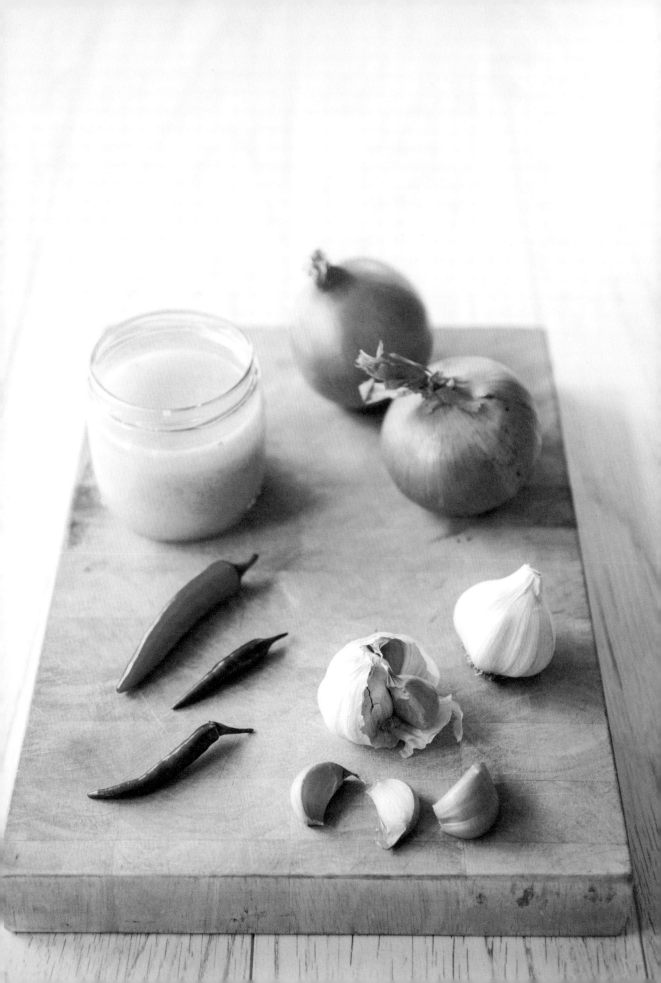

Sage
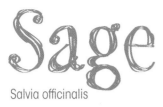

Salvia officinalis

Sof says... Due to the high quantity of thujone in sage, any internal use must be carefully monitored. It should never be used for too long, and never in pregnancy.

Sage is a stalwart of the winter herb garden, delicious for cooking as well as being a great addition to the home remedy cupboard. It has one of the longest histories of medicinal use, known for centuries as a 'cure all'. The Greeks used it for ulcers, and at one point in medieval history it was thought to offer the chance of immortality! The Ancient Chinese used sage to calm nerves and strengthen the digestive system, which it is still used for today; just make a mug of tea with a few leaves to help digest rich food.

Sage is antibacterial, antiviral and antiseptic, so is a good treatment to use on gum infections and mouth ulcers. These same properties also help relieve the symptoms of colds by loosening phlegm and soothing coughs and sore throats. To make a gargle, put a handful of leaves in a mug and pour boiling water over them. Let this sit for five minutes, drain the leaves and leave to cool, then use it to gargle or rinse around your mouth. Add a few drops of peppermint essential oil to this mixture to create a refreshing mouthwash.

Sage tea is often used to reduce the symptoms of excessive sweating and hot flushes at the time of menopause, owing to its active constituent thujone. However, do not take it for too long as it can increase your heart rate and lead to mental confusion. It has been reported to dry up breast milk, so it should not to be used during breastfeeding, and owing to its hormonal effects it should never be used during pregnancy.

sage, witch hazel and rosemary oily skin toner

Sage makes a good toner for oily skin due to its antibacterial and astringent properties. Create your own oily skin toner with sage, witch hazel (to tighten the pores) and rosemary (to increase circulation to dull skin). Also for a lovely smell add either rose essential oil to soothe, or lavender essential oil to cleanse. Apply nightly with cotton wool, although it is important to carry out a skin sensitivity test before using for the first time. Once made up, this skin toner will last for three months.

what you need

- 200ml (7fl oz) still spring water
- 4 tsp (20ml) glycerine
- 2 tsp (10ml) sage tincture
- 1 tsp (5ml) witch hazel tincture
- 1 tsp (5ml) rosemary tincture
- 5 drops of rose essential oil or lavender essential oil

1. Mix all of the above in a bottle.
2. Use nightly with cotton wool.

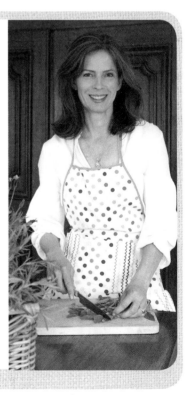

recipe

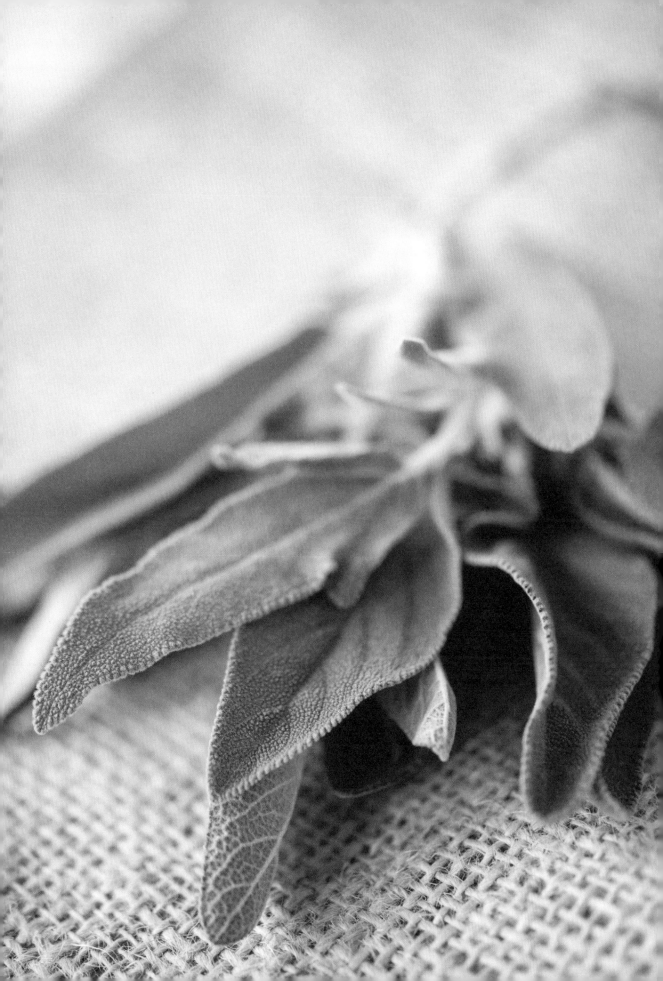

Overindulgence

We've all done it: eaten and drunk too much, with the result that we feel terrible. No more so than at this time of year, so without reaching for the indigestion tablets, which plants can bring relief from this? Here are some suggestions:

VEGETABLE CHARCOAL

This is a herbal remedy that has long been used to correct acidity in the stomach, and to absorb gases and toxins. It also has a mechanical action, stimulating movement of the stomach and intestine, therefore helping to expel whatever is not agreeing with you.

CARBO VEG

Carbo veg is vegetable charcoal in a homeopathic formula, and I have seen it work wonders in cases of indigestion and wind. For example, a patient was complaining of breathlessness, burping with bloat, and general weakness; 20 minutes after a dose of carbo veg he was making a cup of tea, fully recovered.

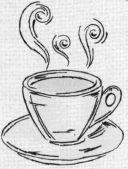

HERBAL TEAS

Mint or chamomile teas both have calming actions on the gut: mint tea tends to revive, while chamomile tea soothes. Also cinnamon and ginger both have good stomach settling actions when used in teas (see their pages for more about these four).

FENNEL

Fennel tea made from the plant's seeds is a favourite to aid digestion; it is particularly good for expelling trapped wind, and for easing indigestion and heartburn. Indeed, fennel is often found in remedies for children's colic. Fennel tea bags are readily available from health food stores, but you can make your own tea by pouring boiling water over a teaspoon of the seeds. Or chew on the seeds to freshen your breath.

The delicate wispy leaves of fennel are a fabulous sight in any garden, especially as they quickly shoot up to tower above all else. Even in winter, their tall hollow stems provide structure to any small herb garden. Fennel is very easy to grow and repeats year after year, needing little maintenance. By late autumn its cheerful yellow flowers are a welcome sight; keep a close eye on them, so come winter you are ready to harvest the seeds. The leaves will bring some of the plant's distinctive flavour to salads.

TUMERIC

This is the spice you will find in your spice rack for adding to curries. It stimulates enzyme production, and due to its strong anti-inflammatory action, it is great for soothing the stomach. The curcumin that gives the spice its strong yellow colour is packed with antioxidants; some even consider this the best natural antioxidant to eat. Tumeric can be used in your cooking or make a tea; just ensure you use a good quality spice, preferably organic.

BROWN RICE WATER

This is a home remedy that will help to rehydrate and replenish the body after a stomach bug. Just put half a cup of organic brown rice in a pan – it will have its all-important outer bran and germ still attached – and cover with double the amount of water you'd normally use for rice. Let the rice cook as usual then drain and keep the water. Let this liquid cool and sip a cup of it to soothe and replenish your gut. You can substitute the rice with barley grains, too.

Arsenic should be used purely as part of the homeopathic remedy arsenicum album, so it is highly diluted and reduced to non-toxic levels. This remedy is never to be made at home under any circumstances.

ARSENIC

Arsenic is probably one of the best-known poisons. But don't panic! I'm not for one moment suggesting you use arsenic to start treating various aches and pains.

As a homeopathic remedy, it is used to treat similar symptoms that arsenic in its crude form would cause: for example, symptoms of acute food poisoning with burning, violent vomiting and diarrhoea. I have taken arsenicum album myself, and it helped me when nothing else would; also, these little white pills are easy to swallow if the thought of taking anything else is just too much.

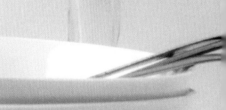

Cinnamon

Cinnamomum

The smell of cinnamon captures the essence of Christmas baking. When I need a winter pick-me-up, I add it to my hot chocolate and am instantly transported to an imaginary Winter Wonderland of alpine cosiness.

Cinnamon is a natural sweetener with a truly distinctive flavour and has traditionally been added to biscuits. It can help with raised blood sugar levels, as it contains an active ingredient thought to mimic insulin, which helps to tell your body it has received something sweet so you don't need more. This helps to avoid the rollercoaster highs and lows that sugar can create. Cinnamon contains antioxidants, making it great to ward off colds. It also has certain antibacterial properties that make it excellent for soothing upset stomachs from overindulgence – very useful at this time of year. If you can't stop thinking about eating yet another mince pie, reach for cinnamon instead to curb your sugar cravings.

The cinnamon we use is the bark of the cinnamon tree, mainly from Sri Lanka and you can buy it in all good supermarkets or health stores. Just add two of the rolled-up sticks to a teapot for a warming mid-morning drink; you won't even need to add honey, as it's naturally sweet. Or if you are in need of a more substantial pick-me-up, put one stick in a pan of milk and slowly simmer so the flavour can infuse the milk, then drink it warm.

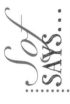 **So SAYS...** Remember sweet woodruff? A spring plant that contains coumarin? Well, some cinnamon contains it too, Cassia or Chinese cinnamon – so don't take too much of it.

ANOTHER FESTIVE SCENT

I love the scent of Christmas trees. I had always assumed this was because of all they promise at this festive time, but it's more than that: pine essential oil has now been shown to be mentally uplifting. Indeed aromatherapists use the oil to treat mild depression and exhaustion, so it is perfect for this busy time of year. You can also add it to a steam inhale to treat winter coughs, but be sure to never take it internally.

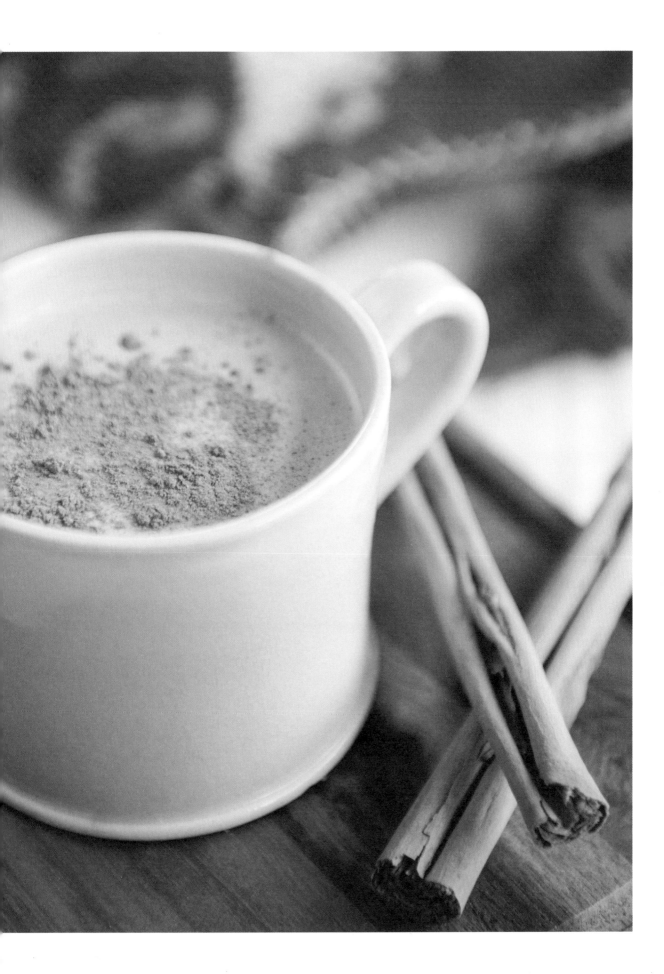

Ginger

Zingiber officinale

This is a great spice rack remedy that originates from the tropics; and it has been used in China for over 3,000 years. The rhizome – a little like a root – of the ginger plant is used, and this is now widely available to buy. Using fresh ginger rhizome is best, and this keeps for several weeks in a cool place. Just peel a chunk of it to make a hot tea, or peel and grate into juices and smoothies to give them a zing. Ginger is fantastic when used with apples, carrots and oranges in a refreshing juice.

USES FOR GINGER

Ginger contains over a dozen antiviral compounds making it excellent for fighting colds; it is also pain relieving, antiseptic and antioxidant, so gargle with ginger and honey to soothe sore throats. Ginger in any form is good for nausea and sickness, taken either as a sweet to suck, biscuits to nibble on, as a tea, or added to a fruit juice. It is also well known for improving circulation, and recent research has found that it may help with arthritis due to the action of its gingerols to reduce pain in joints.

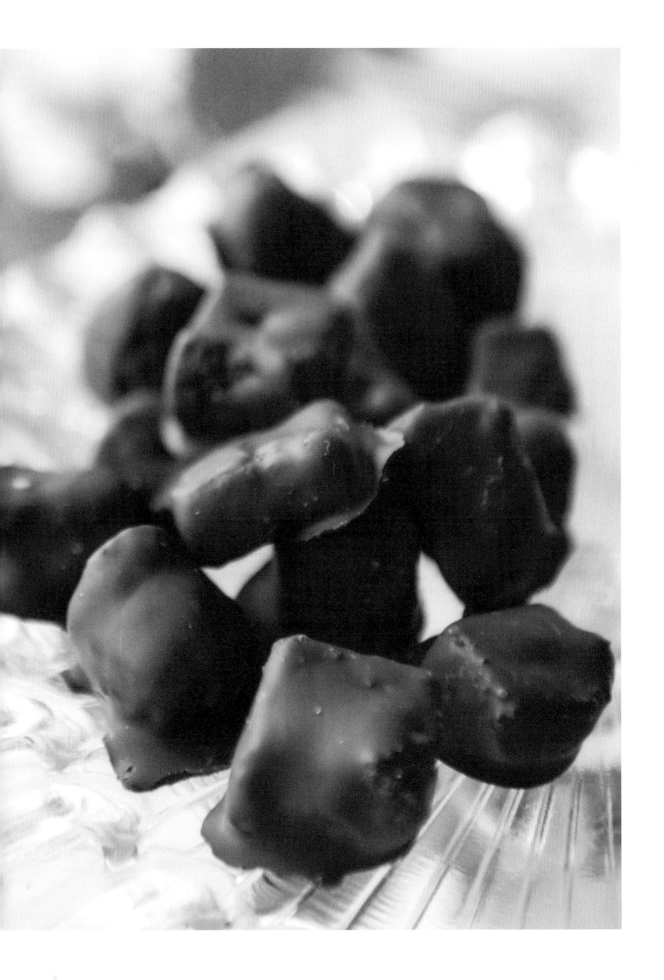

chocolate coated ginger

Have a bit of fun with ginger by trying out this recipe; you will find the crystallized chopped ginger ingredient in the spice or baking section of most food stores. These chocolates will last for up to three months, and make a real after-dinner treat; alternatively, fill a pretty jar with these delicious bites to create some wonderfully tasty Christmas gifts.

what you need

- 150g (5½oz) crystallized chopped ginger
- 2 bars of dark chocolate (70 per cent cocoa solids)
- Clean jam jars and labels
- Metal or wooden skewers, or similar
- Greaseproof (wax) paper

1. Chop up the ginger into smaller pieces, so each piece measures about 1cm (½in) across.

2. Break up the chocolate and melt in a bain-marie (a bowl positioned over a pan of hot simmering water).

3. Once melted, take the chocolate off the heat then dip the ginger into it, several at a time, and fish them out with wooden skewers.

4. Place each chocolate coated piece on the greaseproof paper to dry.

5. Once these are dry, put them in clean, dry jars, label and enjoy.

 Sof SAYS... As these are made with dark chocolate and ginger, they must be good for you!

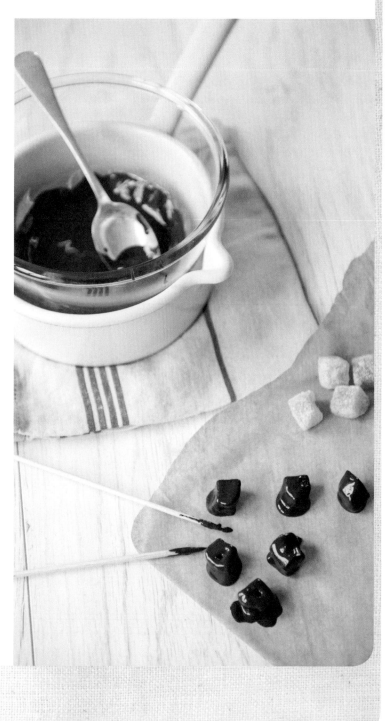

recipe

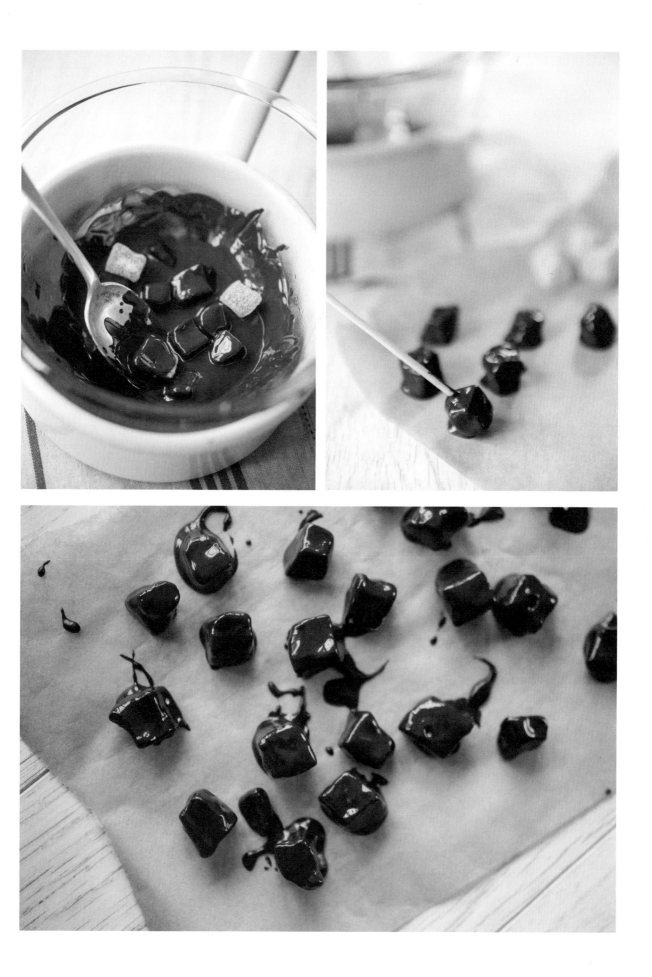

Cloves

Syzygium aromaticum

I always associate the scent of cloves with cosying up and keeping warm in the winter months. Indeed, nothing beats the aroma of cloves in mulled wine, hot chocolate and spiced biscuits to get me in a festive mood. If you like the flavour of cloves, you can use them as a natural preservative in your own cooking; I have used them in my elderberry syrup, but the taste was a little overpowering for me.

Cloves have a numbing effect, which is due to their high content of the natural anaesthetic eugenol; this substance also gives them their distinctive smell. This means that cloves are good for mouth ulcers and toothache; to treat, you can suck on a clove, or dab your ulcer with diluted clove essential oil. This oil is strong, so all you'll need is one drop diluted in 10ml (2 tsp) of sunflower oil.

orange and clove pomander

As fragrant festive decorations, these pomanders really heighten the scent sensation of Christmas, as well as making great presents. To create your own, choose small firm oranges; the bigger looser ones shrivel much more. It can be tempting to cover the orange with just a few cloves, and this looks fine if all you want is a short-term decoration – but it won't last. As we know cloves are a natural preservative, so the more cloves you push into your orange, the longer your pomander will last.

what you need

- 4 small, firm oranges
- 4 handfuls of cloves
- Length of ribbon
- Pen

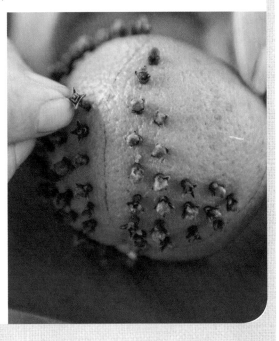

1. To establish where the ribbon will sit, roughly tie it around the orange, mark its position with the pen, then remove it

2. In the space outside the area marked for the ribbon, push the cloves into the orange, covering the entire surface well.

3. Re-tie the ribbon around the orange, then hang it somewhere so you can admire your handy work and enjoy its beautiful scent.

recipe

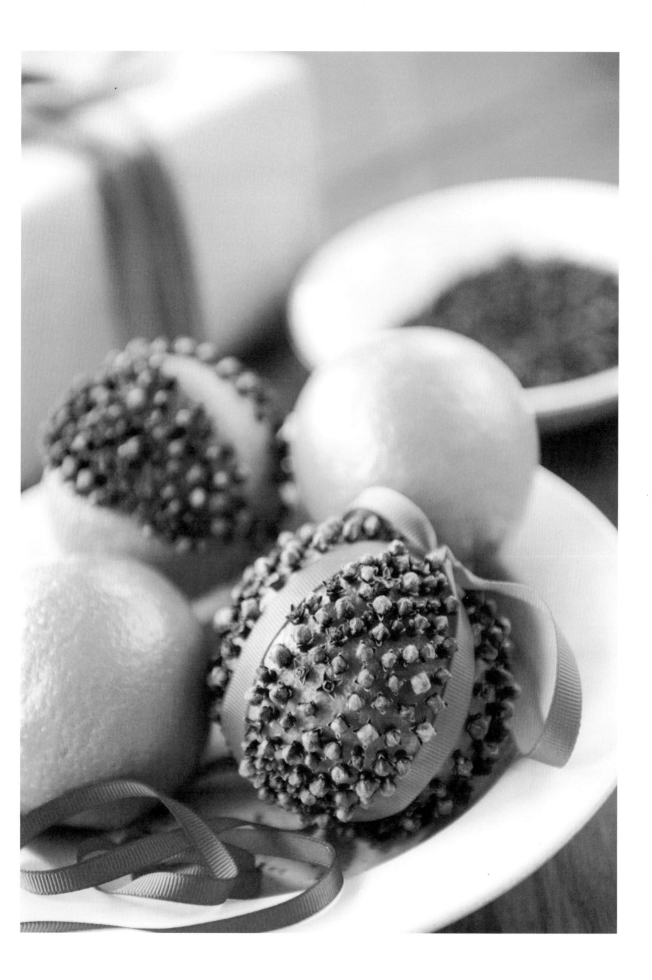

Skincare

In the winter when we spend most of our time wrapped up, it is easy to forget that our skin is our body's largest organ with many vital functions to perform; not least regulating body temperature and indicating any health problems through the appearance of many rashes. Working from the inside to the outside, the skin reflects the hormonal rollercoaster of adolescence with breakouts; and from the outside to the inside, it can absorb much of what you put on it – both good and bad.

NATURAL INGREDIENTS

When you think of the skin in this way it makes sense to carefully consider what you are putting on your own skin. I am not a fan of creams that contain petroleum, paraffin or mineral oil, as these can sit on the skin forming a membrane, acting as a barrier to outside elements. Sometimes this is a good thing – for example, protecting against water and wind. However they can also create a block that prevents the skin from regulating its own moisture, so after a period of use the result can often be that the more of them you apply, the more you need.

The reason these ingredients are commonly added to skin products is twofold: first, their consistency is easy to control, which means they don't melt or harden in warm or cool temperatures; and second, they make cheap additions to these products. I prefer balms and creams that use a mix of oils like cocoa butter, coconut oil and beeswax, all of which contain natural goodies like omegas and vitamins (see Oils).

So SAYS… If you are constantly reaching for your petroleum-based lip balm to treat dry, chapped lips, think again – source a petroleum-free alternative.

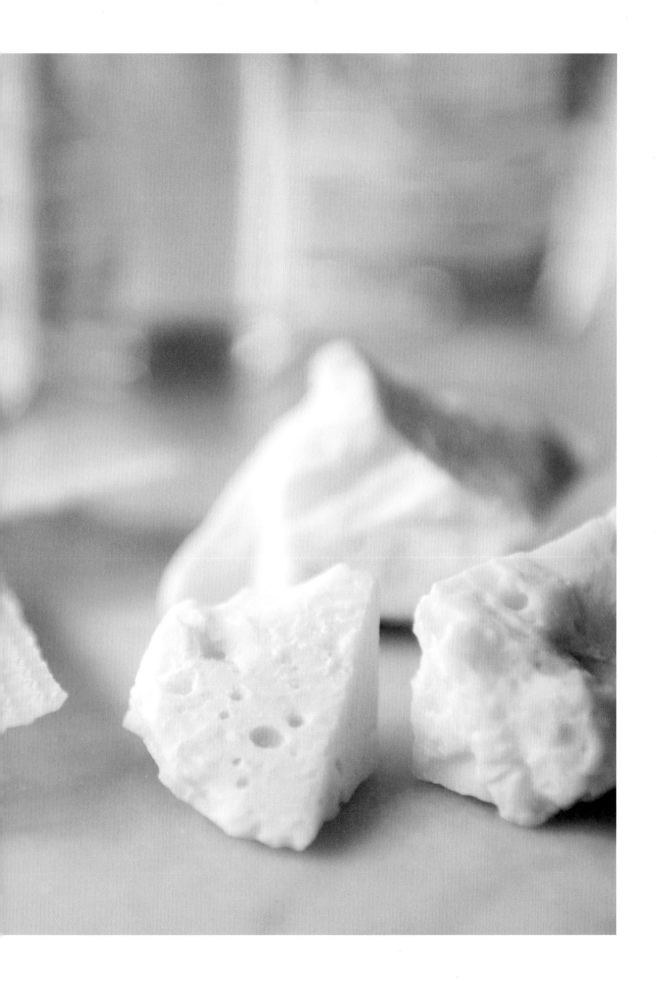

PLANTS AND SKIN

Here is a summary of many of the plants in this book and how they are good for your skin.

For oily skin, several herbs and plants have an astringent and antibacterial action, which make them great for this type of skin:

- **Witch hazel** is one of the best-known astringents; owing to its high tannin and volatile oil content, it makes a great astringent to be used topically.
- **Horsetail** contains the highest level of silica of all known herbs, which makes it excellent for hair and nail care, but also for clarifying the skin. As a great astringent, it tightens pores and helps to stimulate the production of new skin cells.
- **Yarrow** also has an astringent effect, which strengthens skin tone and tightens pores; it also has an antiseptic effect, which is good for healing minor facial cuts.
- **Thyme** has been shown in recent studies to help combat the bacteria that can exasperate acne.
- **Rosemary** is antibacterial so it is good for spots and for lifeless oily skin, as it boosts circulation and elasticity.
- **Rose hip oil** is a dry oil with high levels of omega 3 and 6, which are good for rebalancing large pores. It is the only plant oil that contains a form of vitamin A, which can help with skin problems.
- **Lemon balm** is good for cleansing mildly oily skin, and is also well known for helping to heal cold sores. Its essential oil is very expensive, but lemon balm is a very easy plant to grow and you can make your own tincture from the leaves.

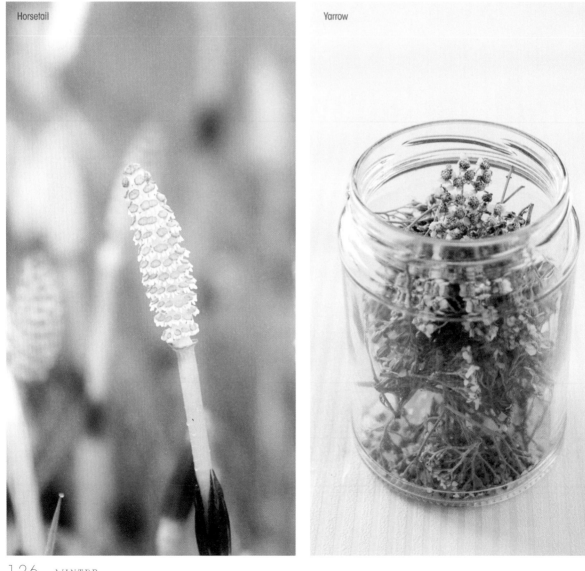

Horsetail

Yarrow

For older skin, try to eat as many fresh fruit and vegetables as possible: most are high in antioxidants, which are good for ageing skin. Other treatments to consider are as follows:

- **Flaxseed oil** – or linseed oil – can be taken internally to boost your levels of omega 3, 6 and 9. It is good for any skin condition, but particularly lifeless, ageing skin. It has a very short shelf life: make sure you don't use rancid oil or you'll be doing yourself no good.
- **Horsetail** is thought to stimulate the production of new skin cells.
- **Rose petal oil** is soothing, restorative and calms dry, red patches.
- **Rose hip oil** is good for older skin as it contains a high level of omega 3; along with omega 6, this assists skin rejuvenation. It soothes, moisturizes and softens fine lines around the eyes as well as scars, and can be taken internally.
- **Ginseng** herb can also be taken internally and can help regulate blood sugar and is antioxidant (please note this does not refer to Siberian ginseng).
- **Horse chestnut** can be applied topically for varicose veins and spider veins due to its high aescin content.
- **Macadamia nut oil** is an excellent fatty oil for dry mature skin, although use it sparingly as it is so fatty.
- **Ginko biloba** is one of the world's oldest trees and is well known for helping memory. For skin it can aid circulation, although it can interfere with medicines, so check before using.

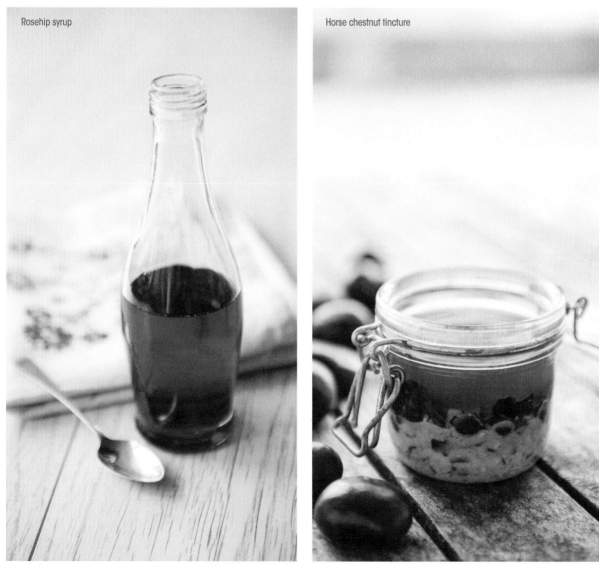

Rosehip syrup

Horse chestnut tincture

Body Scrub

This was one of the first 'potions' I ever made and is incredibly easy; it also makes a great present with the addition of a pretty ribbon and label. Body scrubs are great for reviving dull winter skin: the salt sloughs away dead skin and the oil moisturizes it. Depending on the herbs you use, a body scrub can be invigorating or relaxing. Your herb choice is personal: you can choose ones whose scent you like, or you can choose them for their benefits.

RECIPE OPTIONS

Mint, eucalyptus and rosemary or sage work well together as a winter decongestant body scrub, which is also invigorating and warming.

- The **mint** is a decongestant, refreshing and stimulating.

- The **eucalyptus** is warming, antiseptic, a decongestant and an expectorant

- The **rosemary** is refreshing, stimulating and antiseptic, also helping with nervous exhaustion.

- Or substitute the rosemary with sage for a slightly softer scent.

Alternatively, to make your own unique scrub you could try some other ideas:
- **Marigold** (calendula) makes a healing skin scrub.

- **Lavender or chamomile** creates a relaxing and soothing one. **Honey**, with its natural antibacterial properties, will add an extra element to any body scrub, as well as providing it with a great consistency and smell.

As well as changing the herbs you use, you can also replace the salt with any of the following: sugar, ground almonds, ground oats, ground rice, bran, jojoba exfoliating grains, or apricot kernel powder. The latter two are even, smooth and gentle enough to use on your face.

Sof SAYS... When choosing herbs, be wary of using too much basil or thyme, as the result can leave you with a scrub more suited for use in the kitchen than the bathroom.

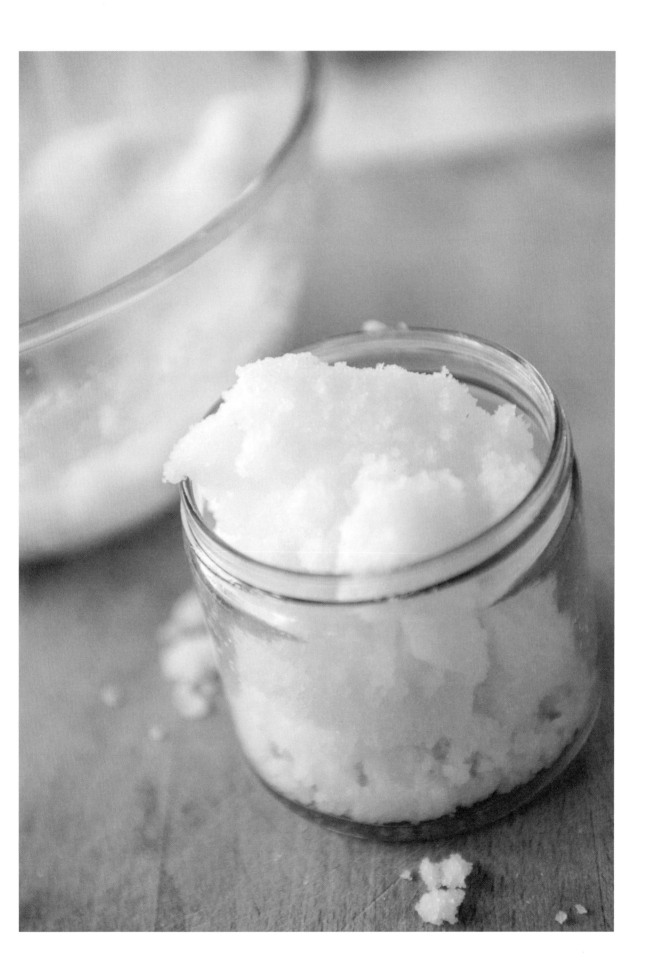

winter body scrub

You can use this as a body scrub or add a spoonful to a hot bath rather like bath salts. However please don't use it if you have sores or cuts, as it will really sting. If you can't find some of the herbs or plants, just add a few drops of their essential oil instead. Or experiment with your own herb combinations.

what you need

To make enough to fill two 300ml (10fl oz) jam jars:
- 600ml (20fl oz) fine sea salt, or enough to fill both your jars
- Approximately 3 sprigs of rosemary, or 20 sage leaves, 30 mint leaves and 20 eucalyptus leaves
- 650ml (1¼ pints) olive or sunflower oil, to fill both your jars plus a little extra
- Pan
- Sieve lined with muslin
- 2 clean jars and labels

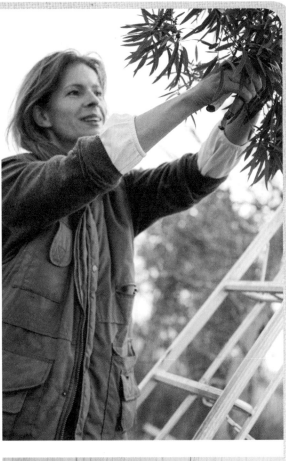

1. Roughly chop the plants and put them in a pan.

2. Cover them with oil and warm them on a very low heat for one hour. Do not even simmer, as the idea is just to warm the contents, encouraging the plants to release some of their goodness into the oil.

3. Line a sieve with muslin and drain the mixture into a bowl, keeping the oil; the leaves can be thrown away.

4. In another bowl pour in your sea salt, then slowly stir the oil into the salt until it reaches a consistency where the salt has completely absorbed all the oil. Keep any left over oil in a jar for later use.

5. Finally, spoon into clean jars and label.

6. This will last for up to one year, though the smell may start to go. Do not use it on any cuts as it will sting.

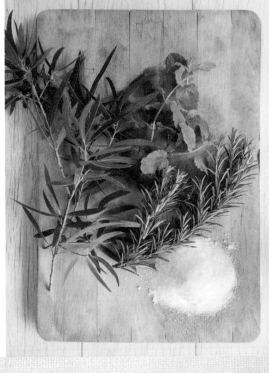

recipe

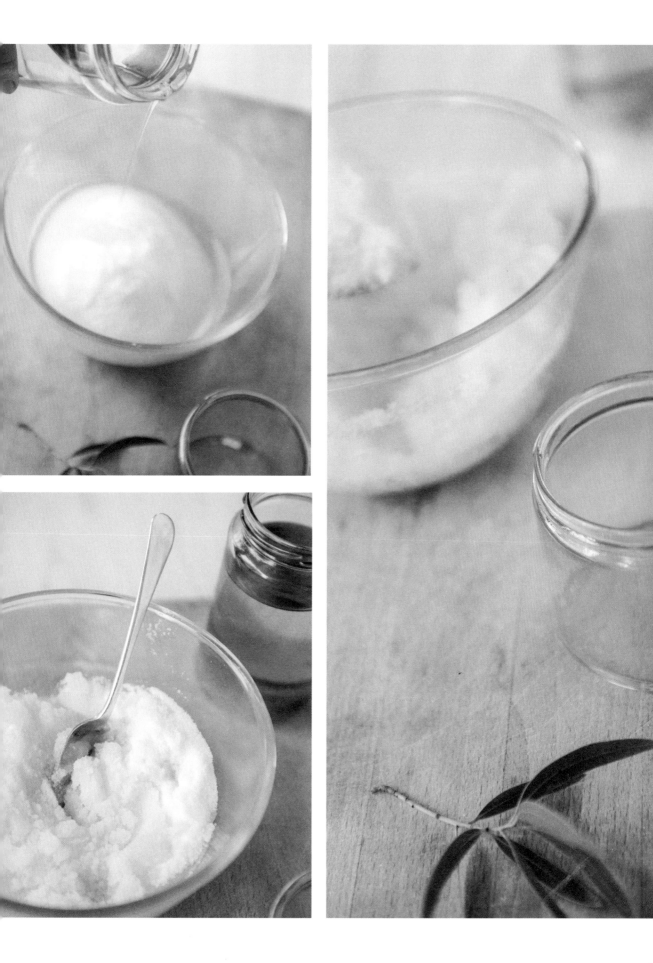

Colds

Winter is often the season we suffer from colds, coughs and numerous viruses. In fact, it is almost inevitable that at some point during these months we will come into contact with one of the 200 or more viruses that cause the common cold.

The main route of infection from external to internal is via our own hands, so the advice to wash them before touching your eyes, nose or mouth makes sense, especially as some viruses can live on inanimate objects – for example, stair handrails – for up to 20 minutes.

There are plenty of alternative natural preventatives and remedies for colds. We have already seen how elderberry can help fight and prevent them (see Elderberries and Elderberry syrup). In addition, there are many excellent homeopathic remedies that can help ease the symptoms of colds: for example aconite, ferrum phos, bryonia and gelsemium. Here are some other remedies and supplements worth considering.

ECHINACEA

Echinacea is the name of a herbal remedy made from this delicate pretty plant of the same name. It works by boosting your immune system with its antiseptic, antiviral and antifungal properties. Studies have shown that it can reduce the length and severity of a cold, as well as your susceptibility to catching them, although long-term use is not recommended.

ZINC

Recent studies have come out in favour of using zinc for colds, finding that it reduces the duration of the average seven-day cold to four days. Zinc has antiviral properties, so start sucking zinc lozenges or taking a good quality zinc supplement as soon as your cold starts. Oysters are a well known source of zinc, and it is also found in other shellfish, fish, red meat, pumpkin seeds and wholegrains.

VITAMIN C

Since 1972, when the Nobel Prize winner Dr Linus Pauling published a paper on the beneficial effects of vitamin C on colds, there have been many studies on the numerous health benefits of this vitamin. Try to consume a good amount of citrus fruits during the winter months, as these are excellent natural sources of this vital vitamin.

PROBIOTICS

Recently the gut has been recognized as playing a large role in the immune system, so keeping it healthy with good natural food is crucial to your overall wellbeing. Probiotics stimulate the growth of micro-organisms with beneficial properties, and these can be found in live natural unsweetened yoghurt or supplements.

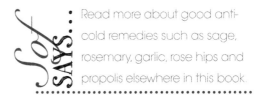 Read more about good anti-cold remedies such as sage, rosemary, garlic, rose hips and propolis elsewhere in this book.

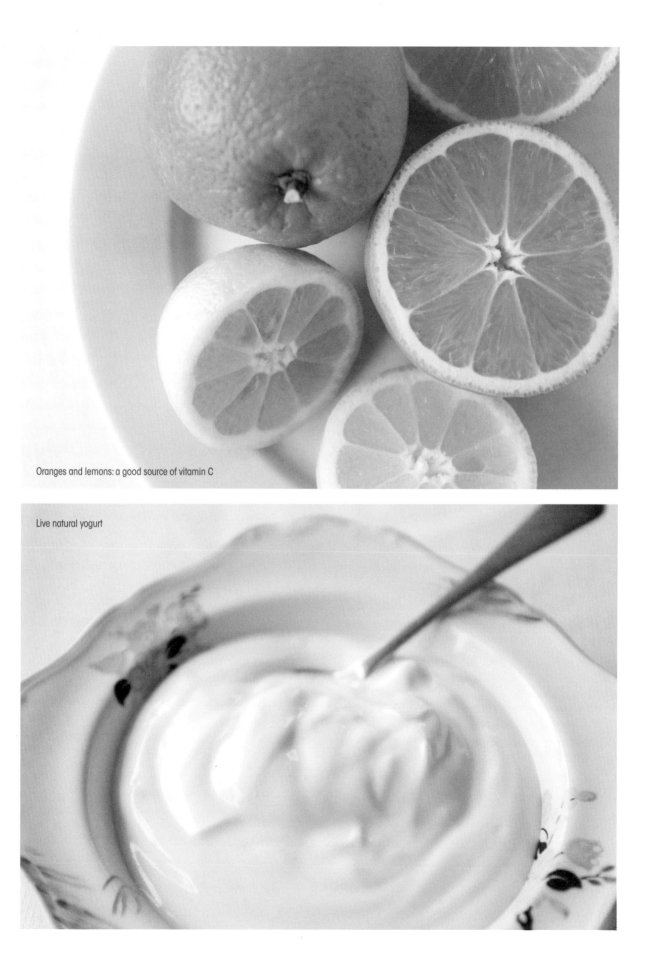

Oranges and lemons: a good source of vitamin C

Live natural yogurt

Bath Time

Nothing beats soaking in a long hot bath on a cold winter night. And now you can add lots of goodies to it, so bathing will be doing you even more good. Throughout this book I've suggested adding various plants to baths to benefit from their properties: chamomile, plantain, rose petals and dandelion flowers.

Another way to use plants in your bath is to make your own bath salts with some essential oil mixed in. These are super easy to make, a jar lasts for ages, and they are all natural with no anti-caking agents or preservatives. Always use real sea salt, as it is full of the rich mineral benefits of the sea and antiseptic. Depending on which essential oil you add, your bath can either be relaxing and calming, or invigorating and uplifting.

Below you will find the recipe for making your own lavender bath salts. However, you might like to try something different. For a muscle soak, add Epsom salts (magnesium sulphate). For an anti-itch soak, just use a tablespoon of bicarbonate of soda (baking soda) neat in the bath; this is particularly good for soothing itchy chicken pox. To clear your winter lungs, add eucalyptus and lavender to the bath salts. And for pure indulgence, add a few drops of rose essential oil to your bath salts for total relaxation.

relaxing lavender bath salts

These bath salts make wonderful presents; even better if you can find pretty old glass jars in which to store them. They are also very easy to make with young children. Be sure to use fine sea salt, as it dissolves more easily in the bath than granular salt. It is often much cheaper to purchase this in bulk from your local health store than in a supermarket; you should also be able to buy lavender sprigs or petals there, too. Lavender essential oil is calming, antiseptic and soothing; a small bottle will go a very long way. Watch out as neat essential oil can sting: if you get it in your eyes, rinse it out with sunflower oil and then water.

what you need

- Fine sea salt to fill your jars
- 10 drops of lavender essential oil per jar
- 1 tbsp lavender petals per jar, or a spring for decoration
- Clean jars and ribbon

1. Decide how many jars you want to make then fill the jars with the fine sea salt.

2. Tip this salt into a bowl and break up any lumps then add about 10 drops of essential oil per jar and stir well, ensuring all the salt has absorbed the oil.

3. If you want add lavender petals sprinkle some in now and stir well.

4. Pour the salt back into the jars and add a sprig for decoration. Label and add ribbons, if making a gift.

5. To use, just add a handful of bath salts to a hot running bath then lie back and relax. Just watch out if you have cuts or sores as the salt will sting.

recipe

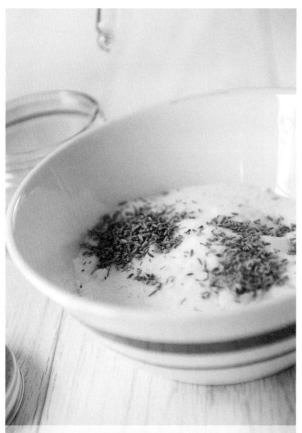

Add essential oil and petals to the salt

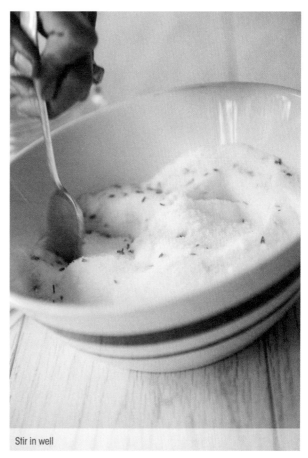

Stir in well

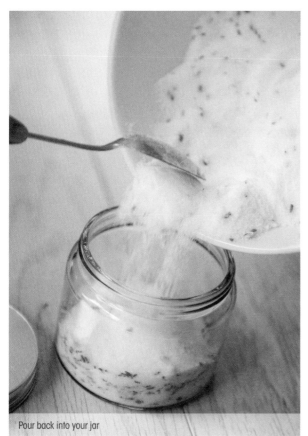

Pour back into your jar

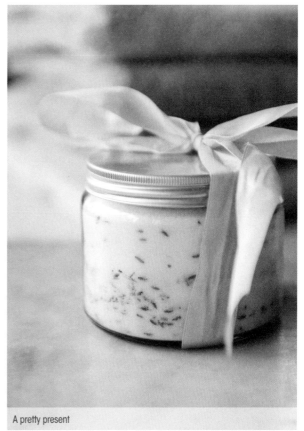

A pretty present

Glossary

A–C

Aescin – the main active compound of Horse Chestnut.

Analgesic – a substance that relieves pain.

Anti-inflammatory – something which when taken or applied (like ice) reduces inflammation.

Antihistamine – this can neutralize the effect of histamine.

Antifungal – inhibits the growth of fungal infections.

Anti-oxidant – found in a variety of fruit and vegetables, beneficial in reducing oxidation (see below) which means they lower the levels of 'free radicals' in the blood, which are thought to contribute to ageing.

Antispasmodic – something that can suppress muscle spasms; a muscle spasm is when a muscle suddenly contracts.

Antiseptic – a substance that kills or prevents the growth of certain micro-organisms and germs, so reducing the possibility of infection and sepsis.

Antibacterial – acts to reduce the growth of bacteria to reduce the possibility of bacterial infection.

Antiviral – acts against viruses to reduce the possibility of viral infection.

Aromatherapy – uses essential oils in the treatment of emotional and physical health concerns.

Astringent – a substance which when applied causes cells to contract.

Carminative – something which eases flatulence.

Compress – a great way to apply treatment externally to a part of the body. see intro on how to make one.

Cordial – a concentrated soft drink, that is diluted with water before drinking. see elderflower cordial.

D–G

Decoction – dried or fresh plant boiled in water for a certain time. see intro on how to make one.

Detox – (shortened form of Detoxification) the process of removing toxins from the body.

Diuretic – something which helps the body release water through increased urination.

Epsom salts – (magnesium sulphate) a mineral compound that has many health benefits (see bruises).

Essential Oil – the natural oil contained within the plant itself, either in the petals, leaves or bark. (see Oils – for more).

Expectorant – encourages the expulsion of phlegm from the lungs.

Flavonoids – a group of compounds that occur naturally in plants, these often are responsible for the plants colour and often have beneficial uses for humans.

Foraging – looking for and using food that often grows wild.

Glycerine – a sweet liquid used in the manufacture of cosmetics and some medicines, like cough syrups and gargles.

H–L

Homeopathy – a form of alternative medicine that was developed by Samuel Hahnemann in the late 18th century, based on the principle of treating 'like with like'.

Histamine – a chemical released during an allergic reaction.

Inflammation – the bodys response to injury or germs, in an attempt to heal itself.

Infusion – this is made by pouring boiling water over your plant material. Like making a tea.

Irritant – a substance that causes irritation.

M–P

Ointment – a fat based liquid for application to the skin.

Omega 3, 6 or 9 – all are essential fatty acids, that are needed for everyday cell function.

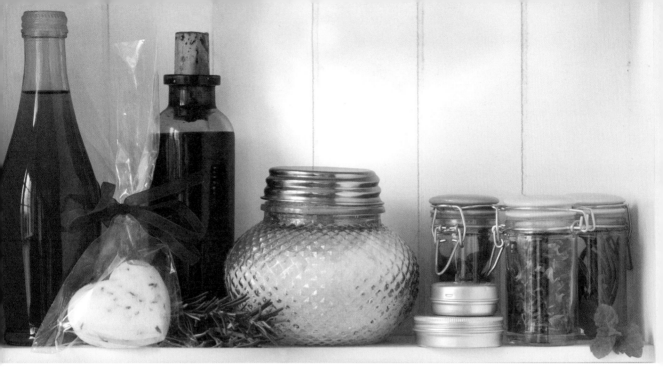

Oxidation – a natural chemical process in our bodies, which releases free-radicals that can damage cells.

Pectin – occurs naturally in most plants, and is used to thicken and gel together jams and jellies. Some plants – apples and citrus fruits have a high amount of pectin. Or you can buy it as a powder to add to your recipes. Some sugars labeled 'Preserving sugar' or 'Jam Sugar' have it already mixed in.

Phytonutrients – nutritional compounds within plants.

Phytochemicals – chemical compounds that occur in plants.

Poultice – a great way to apply treatment externally to a part of the body. Often good for 'drawing out' toxins. see Techniques on how to make one.

Propolis – a substance that bees produce to protect their hives (for more information see Bees in Spring.

Q–Z

Quercetin – a flavonoid that occurs naturally in plants, found in red apples, red onions, berries and tea. It has been found to have anti-inflammatory properties, so it may help with hay fever symptoms.

Rhizome – as in Ginger; it is a swollen underground stem that stores food; roots and shoots come out of this.

Saponins – a group of compounds that occur naturally in plants, they are both water loving (hydrophilic) and fat loving (lipophilic) so are useful in many ways, for example as a foaming agent.

Shrub – a plant that is smaller than a tree and bigger than a bush. So roughly more than 1 metre high and less than 6 metres tall. It also has lots of stems, not just one 'tree trunk'. It can be deciduous or evergreen.

Syrup – a concentrated sugar solution that you can add any flavour to.

Tannins – a group of compounds that occur naturally in plants, that give them their astringent properties. Well known ones occur in tea.

Tincture – plant material soaked in alcohol. see Plantain on how to make one.

Toner – a light liquid that follows cleansing to further cleanse and tighten the skin, prior to moisturising.

Vasoconstrictor – causes constriction of the blood vessels.

Vinegar – a sour liquid consisting of acetic acid, made by fermentation.

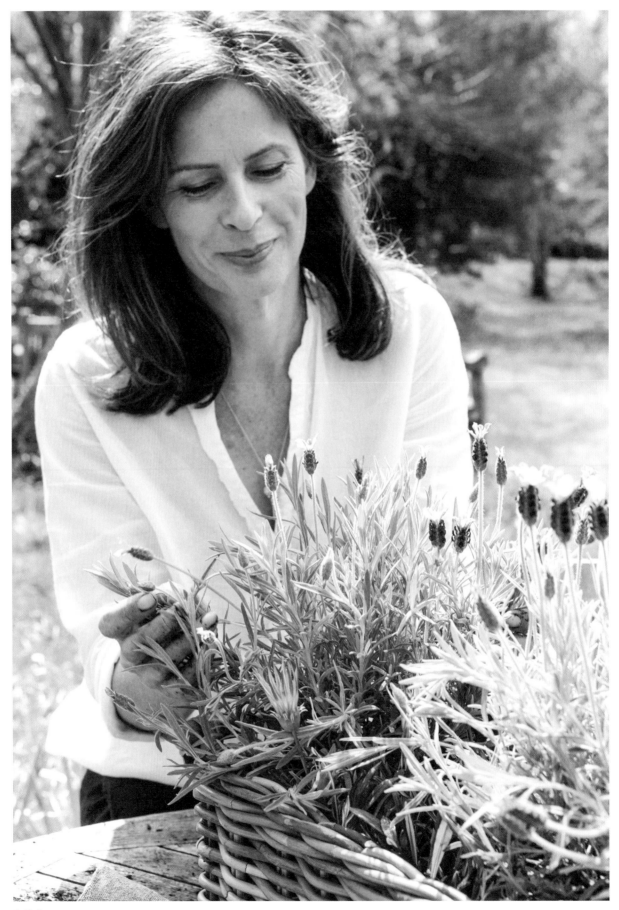

Acknowledgements

This book is the culmination of many years of study, practice and learning, drawing on experts in their field like Aromantics Kolbjorn Borseth, Herbalist Jill Davies, plants woman Jekka McVicar and homeopath Erroll Bowyer, all of whom have been very helpful over the years.

But all this knowledge would not have seen the light of day if not for Verity Graves-Morris, my wonderful Editor, at F&W Media, who approached me with the idea to write this book.

Another editor to thank is Rachel Johnson my first Editor at *The Lady* magazine who encouraged me with her wit and enthusiasm to write my weekly columns all about 'Home Remedies'.

I hope you think this book looks as beautiful as I think it does and that is down to Sarah Clark my designer; along with photographer Jack Kirby from Bang Wallop and Fiona Murray who managed to take some lovely photographs of me on a windy spring day. I would not have found out about Fiona if not for Kirstie Allsopp who has been a wise and practical sounding board over the many years we have been friends, and I am thrilled too that she has written the foreword for this book.

Finally, a huge thanks to all my friends and family for their support, as I try yet another 'white witch' remedy on them. Especially to Charlie and Evie who have definitely been the prime guinea pigs for far too many lotions and potions and odd looking jellies, thank you.

About the author

Sof McVeigh is a mother, writer and founder of The Homemade Company, where the ethos is to bring back the simplicity, joy and sheer fun of making things at home, things that are made with love and full of goodness.

Sof's background as a designer ensures that she really knows how to make things and loves nothing more than tinkering about with paper and glue. After her degree in homeopathy she switched from paper and glue to plants and remedies, leading her to make lotions and potions and all sorts of natural goodies.

Useful Books

The following books I have found useful over the years for references and are invaluable for anyone who wants further information on the many aspects of making your own natural remedies.

GENERAL PLANT AND HERBAL INFORMATION:

The following books have all at some time or other been well thumbed: any book by Jekka McVicar is packed full of information on herbs; Kolbjorn Borseth is the charismatic Scandanavian founder of Aromantics in Scotland and is a great source of knowledge on plants for skin care; Sarah Raven is an English gardener and writer and her new book on wild flowers is one of the most beautiful and informative books I've seen.
For more general gardening advice I love anything by Monty Don, his whole philosophy to gardening is very organic and natural.

Biggs, M., McVicar, J., Flowerdew, B. *The Complete Book of Vegetables Herbs and Fruit.* 2002. Kyle Cathie Limited
Borseth, K. *The Aromatic Guide to the use of Herbs.* 2006. Aromatic Ltd.
Don, M. *The Complete Gardener.* 2003. Dorling Kindersley Limited.
McVicar, J. *New Book of Herbs.* 2002. Dorling Kindersley Limited.
McVicar, J. Jekka's *Complete Herb Book.* (revised edition) 2007. Kyle Cathie Ltd
Raven, S. *Wild Flowers.* 2011. Bloomsbury
Any Collins guide book is invaluable for identification of wild plants – I particularly like the ones with Marjorie Blamey's illustrations, for example: *Collins Pocket guide: Wild Flowers of Britain & Northern Europe,* first published 1974.

A whimsical favourite of mine are any of the '*Flower Fairy*' books, by Cicely Mary Barker, with her beautiful illustrations and the information in them is surprisingly accurate. She was first published in 1923.

MAKING REMEDIES AND DRINKS

In this section Kolbjorn Borseth again is very informative; James Wong has made making remedies very popular in the UK and has his own TV programme; Romney Fraser was the founder of Neals Yard one of the first companies to make herbal and homeopathic remedies easily accessible for all; Andy Hamilton is a British forager and an expert in all things drinkable, his books are very enjoyable to read too.

Borseth, K. *Natural Spa Products.* 2010. Aromatic Ltd.
Borseth, K. *The Aromatic Guide to making your own natural skin, hair and body care products.* 2009. Aromatic Ltd.
Bruton-Seal, J., Seal, M. *Hedgerow Medicine.* 2011. Merlin Unwin Books Ltd.
Fraser, R. *Recipes for Natural Beauty.* 2007. Haldane Mason Ltd.
Hamilton, A. *Booze for Free.* 2011. Transworld Publishers.
Wong, J. *Grow Your Own Drugs.* 2009. HarperCollins Publishers.

NUTRITIONAL AND HOMEOPATHIC INFORMATION

These books are all useful if you want to find out more about what is in the plants and food you are eating.

Matten, G. *The 100 Foods You Should Be Eating.* 2009. New Holland Publishers (UK) Ltd.
Matten, G., Goggins, A. *The Health Delusion.* 2012. Hay House (UK) Ltd.
Murray, M. *Encyclopedia of Nutritional Supplements.* 2001. Three Rivers Press.
Pinnock, D. *Medicinal Cookery.* 2011. Constable and Robinson Ltd.

For very accessible and practical homeopathic advice I always turn to Dr Andrew Lockie's *The family guide to Homeopathy,* published by Hamish Hamilton. Or any book by Neals Yard is also very good on herbs and homeopathy.

Directory

ORGANIC INFORMATION:
UK: Soil association:
www.soilassociation.org

USA: Organic Consumers Association:
www.organicconsumers.org

USA: Rodale Institute:
www.rodaleinstitute.org

GOVERNMENT BODIES:
USA: FDA – government body for safety in drugs in the USA.
www.fda.gov

UK: MHRA – government body for safety in medicines in the UK.
www.mhra.gov.uk

HERBAL AND HOMEOPATHIC ORGANISATIONS:
UK: The National Institute of Medical Herbalists: www.nimh.org.uk

USA: The American Herbalists Guild www.americanherbalistsguild.com

UK: The Society of Homeopaths:
www.homeopathy-soh.org

USA: The American Institute of Homeopathy
www.homeopathyusa.org/

BEES
USA: All about bees:
www.honeybeesuite.com

UK: An interesting take on urban bee keeping in the UK: www.thelondonhoneycompany.co.uk

NATURAL SKINCARE PRODUCTS:
Aromantics: A Scottish based company with some ready made natural products for skincare:
www.aromantic.co.uk

Comvita: New Zealand health Honey products, available in Europe and USA, both in stores and online:
www.comvita.co.uk

ILA: Organic skincare products, with ingredients from all over the world:
www.ila-spa.com

L'Occitane: Natural beauty products, many based on lavender and olive oil. Widely available in Europe in high street stores: www.uk.loccitane.com L'Occitane also has many US stores: usa.loccitane.com

Melvita: European natural organic skincare products , started in France, with organic honey as its basis:
www.uk.melvita.com/organic-beauty-melvita-uk
Melvita has stores throughout Europe and two stores in California and a US website, usa.melvita.com

Neals Yard: One of the first high street herbal and homeopathic suppliers which also stock many great natural skin care products:
www.nealsyardremedies.com

INGREDIENTS
Ainsworth and Helios: Both excellent UK suppliers of homeopathic remedies and creams.
www.ainsworths.com and
www.helios.co.uk

Aromantics: This is Kolbjorn Borseths company (see Useful books) which stock an extensive range of ingredients, all ethically sourced, for you to make your own healthcare products : www.aromantic.co.uk

Bath Bomb Biz and **Just a Soap** are both UK based companies that are great for bath ingredients:
www.bathbomb.biz and
www.justasoap.co.uk

Boiron: The well known French homeopathic company is widely available in the US:
www.boironusa.com

Herbs Hands Healing: Herbalist Jill Davies, based in the UK, supplies many dried herbs, with ready-made herbal preparations and teas www.herbs-hands-healing.co.uk. You can also down load a free E-book by Jill called *Natural Healing and Nutrition*.

Nelsons: A long established UK supplier of homeopathic remedies (since 1860) and is the supplier of Rescue Remedy. It is readily available in the USA too. www.nelsonsnaturalworld.com/en-us

The Homemade Company: This is my company. We sell complete kits for lipbalms, bath bombs and hand balms, so if you are a novice this is the perfect place to start. They also make great presents.
www.thehomemadecompany.com

FORAGING:
It is good to check out people and organisations in your local area. Here are a few ideas to get you started:
USA: Hank Shaw's website:
www.honest-food.net

UK: Andy Hamilton's website:
www.theotherandyhamilton.com

UK: www.foragingcourses.com.

UK: www.selfsufficientish.com

UK: www.gallowaywildfoods.com

Index

acupressure bands 54
aescin 86, 129
air travel 54
allantoin 60
allium cepa 45
aloe vera 55, 90
anti-inflammatories 20, 26, 40, 42, 44–5, 50, 52, 68, 80, 86, 115
antibacterials 22, 40, 52, 64, 68, 70, 78, 108, 110, 112, 126, 128
antidepressants, natural 64, 116
antifungals 64, 78, 108, 110, 132
antihistamines 20, 26, 44–5
antioxidants 20, 40, 82, 98, 108, 115–16, 118, 127, 129
antiseptics 40, 42, 68, 108, 112, 118, 128, 132
antivirals 38, 40, 72, 104, 110, 112, 118, 132
aphrodisiacs 28
arnica 55, 91, 96
arsenic 115
arthritis 26, 118
arundo 45
astringents 42, 68, 104, 112, 126
athlete's foot 64
aucubin 45

balms 14
bath products 15, 52–3, 59, 66–7, 91, 134–5
bees 31, 40
beeswax 40, 62, 124
beetroot 82–3
belladonna 55, 96
betanin 82
bicarbonate of soda 134
blackberry 84, 98–9
blackcurrant 84
blood pressure, high 82, 110
blood sugar balance 116
blood thinners 108
body scrubs 15, 128–31
bone healing 60
borage (starflower) 34–5
bottles 16
brown rice water 115
bruises 55, 91, 96
burn remedies 90, 104
butterflies 31

butters 62

cantharis 90
carbo veg 55, 114
chamomile 52–3, 114, 128
chocolate
    coated ginger 119–21
    lip gloss 28–9
chutney, beetroot, onion and apple 82
cinnamon 114, 116–17
circulation boosters 86, 108, 118, 129
citral 78
citric acid 66
citronella 55
cloves 122–3
cocoa butter 62, 124
coconut oil 124
cold remedies 38, 42, 80, 94, 96, 98, 108, 112, 116, 132–3
cold sore remedies 72, 104, 126
colic remedies 114
comfrey 60–1, 91
compresses 12, 13
conjunctivitis 45, 52
conkers 86–7
cordials 15, 38
cough remedies 38, 92, 108, 116
Culpeper, Nicholas 68
curcumin 115
cystitis remedies 86

damson 84
dandelion 22–3
dandruff 64, 108
decoctions 12
decongestants 38, 110, 112, 128
`detox' herbs 22
digestive aids 22, 50, 52, 55, 70, 78, 108, 114–15, 132
digitalis 96
diuretics 22, 32
drying plants 12, 74–5

earache 54–5
echinacea 132
eczema remedies 26, 32, 34, 42, 52
eggshells, crushed 31
elderberry 92–5
elderflower 38–9
Epsom salts 91, 134

equipment 16–17
eucalyptus 128, 134
euphrasia/eyebright 45
exhaustion 116, 128
expectorant 110, 128
eye conditions 45, 52

fennel tea 114
fever 55, 92, 96
first aid kits, travel 55
flatulence remedies 70, 108, 114
flaxseed oil 127
footbaths 15, 64, 70
foraging 10–11, 30

gallstones 37
gamma linolenic acid (GLA) 34
gardening 10
gargles 15
garlic 110–11
gels 14, 60, 104
ginger 54, 114, 118–21
gingko biloba 127
ginseng 127
glycerine 14
gout 60

haemorrhoids 42, 52, 86, 104
haemostatic agents 42, 68
hair rinses 14, 26, 64, 104, 108
hand balm, mint 72
harvesting plants 74
hawthorn berry 88–9
hay fever remedies 20, 26, 40, 44–5
heart health 88, 96
hedgerow spirit 84–5
homeopathic cocculus 54
homeopathy 11, 45, 54–5, 91–2, 96, 114–15, 132
honey 40–1, 90, 128
horse chestnut 86–7, 127
horsetail 32–3, 126, 127
hydrangea 74–5

immune system boosters 94, 98
infusions 12
insect bite remedies 55, 104
insect repellents 55, 100
ipecac 54
iron, dietary sources 24, 92

itches 20, 59–60, 70, 96, 134

jams 98–9, 156
jars 16
jellies 15, 102–3
joint problems 34, 80, 86, 118
juices, beetroot 82–3

labels 16
labour aids 96
lady's mantle 68–9
lavender 26, 64–7, 70, 128, 134–5
laxatives 22, 91
leather, chewy berry 88
lemon balm 126
lemon verbena 78–9
lip balms 50, 72–3
lip gloss, chocolate 28–9

macadamia nut oil 127
manganese 98
marigold, pot 48–51, 90, 128
memory tonics 108, 129
menopausal symptoms 112
menstrual problems 42, 68
mint 70–3, 114, 128
monkshood (aconite) 54, 96–7
mouthwashes 15, 68, 112
mugwort 100
muscle aches/pains 22, 91, 96, 108,
    134

nail ointment, horsetail 32
nausea remedies 118
nettle, common 24–7
nitrate 82
nosebleeds 42
nux vomica 45

oils 62–3
    essential 16, 59, 116
    infused 12–13, 48–9, 59, 70, 80
ointments 14, 32, 86
omega essential fatty acids 34, 126–7
onion and garlic expectorant 110
orange and clove pomander 122–3
organic produce 30
overindulgence 114–15

painkillers, natural 26, 42, 92, 122

pennyroyal 100
pesticides 40
petroleum-based products 124
phenylethylamine 28
pine essential oil 116
plantain (ribwort) 20–1
poisons 96, 115
pomander, orange and clove 122–3
poultices 12, 13
pre-menstrual tension (PMT) 34
probiotics 132
propolis 40
prostate enlargement 26
psoriasis 32

quercetin 44, 86

raw foods 12, 15
Raynaud's disease 88
relaxation remedies 22, 52, 54, 64, 78,
    108, 134–5
Rescue Remedy 54
rhus tox 91, 96
ringworm remedies 64
rose 56–9, 127, 134
rose hip 80–1, 126, 127
rosemary 100, 108–9, 112, 126, 128
rowan berry 102–3
ruta 91

sabadilla 45
sage 100, 112–13, 128
salads 15, 36, 82
salicylic acid 42, 92
sambucus 92
scarring 34
sedatives 52
shock, remedies for 96
silica 32, 126
skin 34
    dry 20, 50, 59, 68, 129
    oily 26, 38, 42, 108, 112, 126
    older 127
    renewal 32, 60, 126–7
    sensitive 26, 50
    toners 14, 68, 70, 86, 112, 126
    tonics 22
    winter care 124–31
sloe 84
slugs and snails 31

soil 30
sore throat remedies 38, 112, 118
soups 15, 24–5, 36, 82
southernwood 100
spot remedies 104, 126
steam inhalations 108–9
sterilization 16
stings 20, 55
sugar cravings 116
sunburn remedies 55, 59, 64, 90
supplements 11
sweet woodruff 37
syrups 15, 80–1, 92, 94–5, 127

tansey 100
teas, herbal 12, 22, 52, 78, 112, 114
thread veins 86, 129
thyme 126
tinctures 12, 20, 86–7, 127
toothache 122
travel 54–5
turmeric 115

ulcers
    leg 60
    mouth 52, 112, 122

Valentine's day 28–9
varicose veins 42, 52, 60, 86, 104, 129
vegetable charcoal 55, 114
vertigo 54
vinegars 12, 90
vitamin A 22
vitamin C 80, 84, 92, 132

wart remedies 31
waxes 62
witch hazel 90, 91, 104–5, 112, 126
wood sorrel 36
wormwood 100–1
wound healing 20, 22, 40, 42, 60, 64,
    68
wyethia 45

yarrow 42–3, 92, 126

zinc 132

A DAVID & CHARLES BOOK
© F&W Media International, Ltd 2013

David & Charles is an imprint of F&W Media International, Ltd
Brunel House, Forde Close, Newton Abbot, TQ12 4PU, UK

F&W Media International, Ltd is a subsidiary of F+W Media, Inc
10151 Carver Road, Suite #200, Blue Ash, OH 45242, USA

Text and Designs © Sof McVeigh 2013
Layout and Photography © F&W Media International, Ltd 2013, except pages 4, 5, 18, 19, 23,
33, 35, 36, 37, 39, 45, 46, 47, 54, 55, 69, 76, 77, 93, 97, 106, 107, 114, 115 © iStockphoto
Photography on pages 7, 8, 11, 30, 64, 138 by Fiona Murray
Illustrations © Sarah Clark

First published in the UK and USA in 2013

Some source material has previously been publsihed in *The Lady* magazine.

The author and publisher have made every effort to ensure that all the instructions in the book
are accurate and safe, and therefore cannot accept liability for any resulting injury, damage or
loss to persons or property, however it may arise.

Names of manufacturers and product ranges are provided for the information of readers, with
no intention to infringe copyright or trademarks.

Metric and imperial measurements are given for the recipes in this book. Use one set of
measurements only, not a mixture of both.

A catalogue record for this book is available from the British Library

ISBN-13: 978-1-4463-0318-4 paperback
ISBN-10: 1-4463-0318-7 paperback

Printed in China by RR Donnelley for:
F&W Media International, Ltd
Brunel House, Forde Close, Newton Abbot, TQ12 4PU, UK

10 9 8 7 6 5 4 3 2 1

Publisher: Alison Myer
Junior Acquisitions Editor: Verity Graves-Morris
Project Editor: Freya Dangerfield
Proofreader: Beth Dymond
Design Manager: Sarah Clark
Photographer: Jack Kirby
Senior Production Controller: Kelly Smith

F+W Media publishes high quality books on a wide range of subjects.
For more great book ideas visit: www.stitchcraftcreate.co.uk